Tips & TimeSavers
for
Home Health Nurses

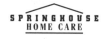

SPRINGHOUSE
HOME CARE

Springhouse Corporation
Springhouse, Pennsylvania

Staff

Executive Director
Matthew Cahill

Art Director
John Hubbard

Managing Editor
David Moreau

Acquisitions Editors
Patricia Kardish Fischer, RN, BSN; Louise Quinn

Clinical Consultants
Maryann Foley, RN, BSN; Collette Bishop Hendler, RN, CCRN

Senior Editor
Michael Shaw

Copy Editors
Cynthia C. Breuninger (manager), Karen C. Comerford, Christine Cunniffe, Brenna H. Mayer

Designers
Arlene Putterman (associate art director), Joseph Clark, Jacalyn Facciolo

Production Coordinator
Margaret A. Rastiello

Editorial Assistants
Beverly Lane, Mary Madden

Manufacturing
Deborah Meiris (director), Pat Dorshaw (manager), T.A. Landis

Indexer
Barbara Hodgson

Printed in the United States of America.
TTHHN-010397

Ⓡ A member of the Reed Elsevier plc group

Library of Congress Cataloging-in-Publication Data
Tips and timesavers for home health nurses
   p. cm.
   Includes index.
1. Home nursing—Handbooks, manuals, etc.
2. Nurses—time management—handbooks, manuals, etc.
I. Springhouse Corporation
[DNLM: 1. Home nursing-handbooks]
DNLM/DLC   97-65380
ISBN: 0-87434-917-6   CIP

Contents

Foreword

Home care is now the fastest growing segment of the health care delivery system. Working in patient's homes and local communities, nurses are tackling clinical challenges that not long ago were the sole domain of hospital practice. Home care will continue to be a major source of opportunity for nurses as the profession advances into the next century.

The ability to improvise equipment and to respond to unexpected events at a moment's notice have long been essential skills for home care nurses. In today's managed care environment, the need to think quickly and creatively is becoming even more intense. Cost-conscious managed care organizations are reducing the number of visits allowed to accomplish clinical goals. To help clients remain independent in the community, home care nurses must work smarter at every turn.

Under these conditions, home care nurses need a how-to book to help them become more efficient, creative, and cost-effective. In light of the fast pace of contemporary practice, pointed tips and advice are more useful than lengthy text. That's why *Tips and TimeSavers for Home Health Nurses* is the perfect resource to help you succeed in today's exciting but high-pressure work environment. This unique nursing tool is concise, lively, and eminently readable.

It's easy to locate information related to your professional needs and clinical concerns inside *Tips and TimeSavers for Home Health Nurses*. Six chapters cover major activities of home care nursing: the home visit, assessment, patient teaching, medications, I.V. therapy, and procedures. Four chapters cover major client populations: adult, geriatric, pediatric, and maternal-neonatal. There's also a chapter on nursing law. Each chapter is divided into helpful subtopics and each tip or timesaver is titled in boldfaced text.

Within each chapter, you'll find secrets for improvising equipment, creative ways to enhance your patient's quality of life, and field-tested techniques to eliminate health care hassles. The variety of topics covered is simply amazing: rapid assessment techniques, supervision of home health aides, care for caregivers, ingenious medication reminders, ostomy care tips, cost-saving comfort measures, creative teaching strategies, documentation pointers, diabetes care tips, risk reduction for geriatric patients, play therapy for pediatric patients, and much more. Most important, advice is based on the practical experiences of nurses who confront the realities of providing home care every day.

I have practiced for more than 20 years in home care nursing. Like many of my colleagues, I pride myself on being able to overcome clinical challenges with little more than the tools available at home. However, by reading *Tips and TimeSavers for Home Health Nurses*, I learned many creative new ways to deal with clinical problems. I found innovative ideas in every chapter. *Tips and TimeSavers for Home Health Nurses* is an invaluable reference for the experienced home care nurse and should be required reading for nurses new to home care as well as students just now embarking on a nursing career.

Paula Milone-Nuzzo, RN, PhD
Associate Professor
Chair, Specialty Care and
   Management Division
Yale University School of Nursing

1

The Home Visit

Contents

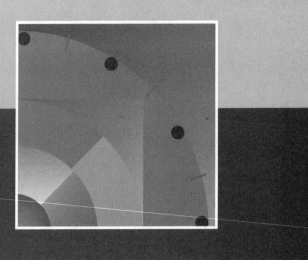

Contributors

The following nurses provided tips and timesavers for this chapter:

Dianne Charron, RN, BSN

Jill Dailer, RN, BSN

M. Dolan, RN

Carla Goodmurphy, RN, OCN

Mona Jacob, RN

Leah McNulty, RN, BSN

Angie Perry, RN

Lynn Nelson, RN

Making home visits

BETTER BUSINESS

Are you, as I am, dealing regularly with managed care organizations? Then check out these tips, which have helped me balance patients' needs with big businesses' efficiencies:
• Remember that managed care is about cost efficiency. So keep your clinical skills up-to-date, and stay abreast of new treatment strategies and new methods for educating patients.
• Always document successful patient outcomes, and be sure to note efficient and effective interventions.
• Become familiar with community resources that can help your patients achieve more independence.
• Find out how your agency communicates with managed care organizations; suggest improvements wherever possible. And work within your agency to resolve problems.
• Learn as much as possible about payment trends for health care, types of managed care organizations, and your agency's strategies for working with the various organizations.
• Accept that managed care is here to stay, at least until something else comes along.

DISQUALIFIED

When reviewing my patient's eligibility for home care under Medicare, I'm on the lookout for these disqualifiers:
• Patient leaves home frequently for social activities.
• Patient drives a car.
• Patient goes to adult day-care for nonmedical reasons.
• Patient routinely goes to a relative's home.
• Patient regularly shops for groceries or goes out for other business.
• Patient stays home because of insecurity, fear, or other "nonmedical" reason.

HOMEBOUND OR NOT?

Some of my patients ask about qualifying for Medicare reimbursement for home care services. I respond by explaining

these eligibility criteria, which must be met:
• Patient can't leave home.
• Patient leaves home with considerable difficulty and great effort.
• Patient leaves home infrequently and then only for a short time.
• Patient leaves home to receive medical care only.

STREET SMARTS
Need a new street map of your agency's service area? In my territory, you can find local maps at most bookstores, pharmacies, and convenience stores. Sometimes, real estate agencies are good sources of maps, too. Why not check them out?

MAP SKILLS
It wasn't until I became a home health nurse that I learned to really appreciate maps—they're one of the most important items in a nurse's bag of tricks. And I'm willing to share my secret:

When buying a map, be sure to get one with plenty of detail, even if you have to pay more. Then, bone up on your map-reading skills, and study the map until you can tell at a glance whether you're heading north, south, east, or west. Use your map and new skills to plan out a route before you get into your car and start driving.

MARKED MAP
As a home care nurse, I sometimes have trouble finding a patient's address when I'm unfamiliar with the area. So I cut a city map into 8" × 12" (20 × 30 cm) sections. I put two sections back to back, laminate both sides, and seal the edges. Each morning, I draw my route in erasable marker on the plastic-coated map. This provides an easy-to-handle, visible reference that is especially valuable when I'm driving in heavy traffic.

Managing time wisely

HELPFUL HINTS: EASY AS A TO Z

I keep a pocket-sized address book with me and use it to jot down any helpful information—such as new drugs or doctors' names and specialties. Because my entries are in alphabetical order, I can quickly find what I'm looking for.

TACKLING ORGANIZATION

As a home health care nurse, I use a tackle box to keep my venipuncture supplies organized. The box's small compartments and carrying handle are great conveniences.

DISK-ADVANTAGE

As a home health care nurse, I frequently need more equipment than I like to carry with me. For instance, when measuring the size of lesions or decubitus ulcers, I find the tip of my finger not exact enough but rulers too bulky *and* breakable.

My solution is to carry a measurement disk made for reading the results of intradermal skin tests. It's accurate and easy to carry. If the disks aren't available at the home health agency, I can get a supply simply by writing to the drug companies that manufacture the skin tests.

CALLING CARDS

During my home health care visits, I found that patients and their families often forgot scheduled appointment times and so weren't home when I arrived.

To avoid this, I started giving patients and their family my business card with the next appointment written on the back. This way, they had a reminder as well as the agency's phone number if they needed to call.

Keeping safe

SAFE MOVES

In some neighborhoods and homes, I feel uneasy, kind of scared. Rather than leave things to luck, I take these steps to help ensure my safety:
• Verify where my patient lives and call the family to confirm my visit before I leave the agency.
• Leave a copy of my itinerary at the agency.
• Plan my visit for early in the day and bring a nurse "buddy" along if the patient lives in an unsafe area.
• Wear business clothes and a name tag, and carry agency identification since I don't wear a uniform.

PREVENTING LOCKOUTS

This may sound silly, but it's happened to me more than once: I've locked myself out of my car. To prevent such situations from becoming safety issues (not to mention major time-wasters), I now carry an extra set of keys and enough money for emergency transportation and phone calls. In my pocket, I also keep a list of important phone numbers, such as police and fire departments and, of course, my agency.

ON THE ROAD

Three winters ago, I was stranded for 2 ½ hours on a lonely stretch of road. The reason: My car had run out of gas (it was dumb of me not to have checked the gauge before I left the agency). Waiting for help wasn't much fun, but I learned a lesson. Here's what I do now to help make sure I won't be left in the lurch again:
• Take my car for tune-ups and other routine service so it runs well.
• Check the car's gas gauge to be sure the tank's full before leaving for a home visit.
• Allow extra travel time in bad weather.

• Keep a flashlight, blanket, and snacks handy.
• Carry a shovel, sand, antifreeze, dry gas, coolant, and jumper cables in the trunk.

By the way, I also joined an automobile club so I can have quick access to road service.

TIME TO LEAVE

I've been a home care nurse for more than 10 years, and I don't panic easily. But a recent incident in a patient's home frightened me. Since then I think more about my safety and ask myself these questions as soon as I enter a home:
• Where are the exits?
• Does anyone appear to be under the influence of alcohol or drugs?
• Can I treat my patient quickly?

If the situation seems risky, I leave immediately.

BEAT THE HEAT

During the summer, I keep a bottle of frozen drinking water with me when I make home visits. The frozen bottle keeps other refreshments cold and, as it thaws, provides my patients and me with cool water—a lifesaver in a heat wave or emergency.

Keeping patients safe

USER-FRIENDLY LIVING ROOMS

In many of my patients' homes, the living room is a gathering place for friends and relatives, a center of social activity. Unfortunately, few of the rooms are user-friendly to home-bound patients. So, as soon as I can, I talk with the family about making some changes. These are the things I suggest most often:
• Replace thick or shag carpet with low-pile carpet, or cover the carpet with low-pile area rugs to make walking or using a wheelchair easier.

• Put a cushion on an easy chair if the patient has trouble getting out of a low seat.
• Install handrails along walls.
• Arrange furniture along walls; open areas are easier to move around in.
• Place a telephone within easy reach; that may mean attaching a longer wall cord or installing a cordless phone.
• Move all wires (both electrical and telephone) so no one trips on them.

BETTER REST

My immobile patients as well as many of those on the mend from surgery or illness are not only homebound, but bedroom bound. To improve their safety, comfort, and quality of life, I make these recommendations to the family:
• Rent or buy a hospital-style bed with side rails and attached trapeze.
• Raise a regular bed (on 4 × 4 blocks) about 4" (10 cm) to make it the same height as a wheelchair.
• Lock or remove wheels or casters on the bed.
• Position one side of the bed against a wall, to keep it stationary.
• Place a commode chair, urinal, or bedpan close to the bed.
• Arrange furniture so the patient can look out a window.
• Place a telephone near the bed.
• Provide a night-light.
• Keep a flashlight and extra batteries near the bed.

EMERGENCY NUMBERS

During my initial home health care visit, I give my patient a list that includes my agency's daytime and after-hours phone numbers in large, bold print; the agency's nursing specialties; the names of the specialty nurses; and the name and phone number of the patient's doctor. When posted on the refrigerator or near the phone, the list becomes a handy resource for the patient and family.

HOME CARE HELPER

When a bedridden, chronically ill patient returns home, I encourage the family to buy or rent an inexpensive, portable intercom—one like a baby's monitor, to be specific—then place it in the patient's bedroom. The intercom allows the family to move about the house and still hear the patient's requests for assistance.

Dealing with families

SPIRITUAL COMFORT

Occasionally, a patient and family ask for my help in arranging religious rituals. If I think it's appropriate, I pray with them, even if they are of another faith. To me, all basic spiritual questions and needs are the same, despite different rituals, languages, and customs.

Still, I'm always careful not to impose my own prayers. Instead, I try to reinforce the spiritual things—a love for reading or music, for example—that have sustained the family during other difficult times. Of most importance, I let them know I'm there to help; people in spiritual pain need understanding, not preaching.

DEALING WITH GRIEF

Confronting the death of a spouse or another loved one is a lonely experience. I try to help the bereaved person cope in the following ways:

• Explain that, initially, feelings of denial and disorientation predominate; these feelings temporarily cushion the sense of loss while the bereaved person tries to accept that death has really occurred. I caution that, eventually, the bereaved must face grief to recover from the loss.

• Reassure the bereaved person that, after denial, the emotions of sadness, guilt, anger, and even hatred are normal. I stress the importance of sharing these emotions with someone.

• Refer a bereaved spouse to community agencies for guidance and temporary assistance with legal and financial issues.

RECOGNIZING AND AVOIDING BURNOUT

Many of my patients have chronic or terminal illnesses, and their immediate caregivers, who are usually family members and on duty for 24 hours a day, 7 days a week, are vulnerable to stress and burnout. To help caregivers minimize their stress, I suggest they try one or all of the following:

• Take up a new hobby or revive interest in a favorite one.
• Eat a balanced diet and get adequate rest.
• Practice progressive muscle relaxation.
• Experiment with guided imagery.
• Learn to meditate.
• Read funny books, watch comedies, and try laughing at your own mistakes.
• Pray often or whenever you feel the need.
• Set priorities.
• Delegate some tasks to others.

CARING AFTER DEATH

Nurses at Hospice Nana in Bristol, N.H., don't stop caring after one of their patients dies. Instead, they make bereavement visits to the family 1, 2, and 3 weeks after the patient's death, then at 3 months, 6 months, and 1 year. They also visit at other times if they think the family needs it.

The hospice nurses have found that many families experience health-related problems within 6 months after a patient's death. That's when the cards have stopped coming, visits from friends have become less frequent, and the death is supposed to be "a thing of the past." Family members, whose time had been consumed by caring for the terminally ill person, may find they now have long hours of unfilled time. The loneliness may be difficult to bear. They may become depressed and predisposed to illness.

The visits have helped the nurses offset the loneliness and detect illnesses early. They have, for instance, detected hypertension that developed in a widow 6 months after her hus-

band died and severe depression in a mother whose child
died of leukemia.

The nurses welcome the chance to support the family
throughout the year following the patient's death—and families welcome the support and preventive health care they
receive.

Working with home health aides

ELIGIBILITY FOR A HOME HEALTH AIDE

Some of my patients require more care than their caregiver
spouses or families can realistically provide. When that's the
case (and it often is when a patient and spouse are elderly), I
request the assistance of a home health aide (HHA).
Medicare will cover the HHA's visits under these circumstances:
• The HHA is considered a secondary service.
• There's already a skilled service, such as nursing or physical
therapy, in the home.
• There's a plan of care that identifies care by the HHA as reasonable and necessary.
• A doctor's order specifies the type and frequency of care.
• The HHA is qualified to provide personal care and does so
to attain or maintain the patient's health or to facilitate treat-
ment of an illness or injury.
• The HHA visits the home on a part-time or intermittent
basis.
• Every 14 days, a registered nurse supervises the care given by
the HHA.

EASY DIRECT SUPERVISION

In my 3 years as a home health nurse, I've supervised several
home health aides (HHAs), checking on each HHA every 14
days as required. To be sure my evaluation of the HHA is
complete, I prepare a detailed but simple questionnaire
before making the supervisory visit. The questionnaire

includes rankings (from poor to excellent) that I can easily mark during or after the observation. Areas I evaluate include:
• the physical care given to the patient
• the care provided compared with the documented care plan
• the reasonableness, necessity, and appropriateness of the care to my patient's health needs.

PROVIDING FEEDBACK
Whenever I supervise a home health aide (HHA), I like to provide two types of feedback: (1) direct, which is my own observation, and (2) indirect, which consists of comments from the patient. (Few patients are willing to discuss an HHA's performance when the HHA is present.) Comments I seek for the indirect evaluation include:
• the patient's general satisfaction with the HHA: performance, punctuality, manners
• the patient's response to the HHA's care.

   I also ask the patient to describe any changes in his condition or care that I might not have observed.

2

Assessment

Contents

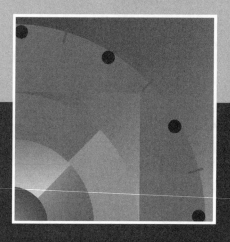

Contributors

The following nurses and health care providers contributed tips and timesavers for this chapter:

Linda Graves Allen, RN, BSN	Dorothy M. Kellogg, RN
F. Kate Davis, RN	Diane Klaiber, RN
Barbara Engram, RN, MSN	Nancy Kunz, RN
Pat Elswick, RN	Frances Marshall, RN
Elizabeth A. Hendrix, RN, BSN	E. Jane Mezzanotte, RN, MSN
Beatrice Humphris, RN	Christine Ozoro, RN, BSN
Lisa Inman, BSN	Patti Shewbart-Llewellyn, RN
Stephen M. Keller, EMT	Melissa A. White, RN, BSN

Obtaining the health history

NURSING HISTORY HELPER

To help remember all the pertinent information I need for taking a complete, systematic nursing history, I use a pocket-sized card as a guide. Here's how to make one for yourself:

First, list the categories you wish to include, such as:
• vital statistics
• patient's understanding of illness
• patient's expectations
• social and cultural history
• significant data.

Then type these subjects, with questions or specific items to ask the patient about, on both sides of a 5" × 7" (13 × 18 cm) card. Take the card to a local printer and have it reduced in size (to about 3" × 5" [8 × 13 cm]) and laminated to withstand the wear and tear of daily use.

The card is handy and easy to use, and it will last for years.

EYE TO EYE

My agency's clientele includes a number of patients who have dementia. When I need answers from those patients, here's how I handle the situation:

First, I establish eye contact to hold the patient's attention and help the patient focus on what I'm saying. Then, I ask specific questions that call for limited responses, such as "Do you have pain in your legs?" I avoid using pronouns. Instead, I address the patient by name. If I'm talking about someone else, I use that person's given name.

LEADING QUESTIONS

When I first started interviewing patients about their health history, it didn't take me long to discover an interesting fact: the information I'd collected wasn't complete. Then a colleague suggested I might be asking leading questions that elicited "correct" answers.

Now I'm more careful about wording questions. For example, I avoid saying "You don't use I.V. drugs, do you?" because such a question will almost always get a "no" response whether the patient uses drugs or not. Instead, I simply ask, "Do you use I.V. drugs?" The results of my newly worded questions: health histories with more information.

DESCRIBING DYSPNEA

In recent months, I've interviewed several patients about their dyspnea, and I've come to realize that what one person considers severe shortness of breath, another considers mild. So to make my assessments as objective as possible, I now ask patients to describe briefly how various activities, such as walking, climbing stairs, and carrying groceries, affect their dyspnea.

RECOGNIZING DEPRESSION

Depression's not uncommon in my once-active patients who are now ill. If I suspect a patient is depressed, I ask him (and the caregiver) these questions:
• Has your appetite changed or have you recently lost or gained weight for no explainable reason?
• Do you have difficulty sleeping or do you sleep more than usual?
• Have you withdrawn from friends and family? How about social activities?
• Do you become agitated easily? Do you explode into angry outburst for no apparent reason?
• Have you lost interest in taking care of yourself?
• Do you feel your life is worthless?
• Do you feel helpless or as though you are in other people's way?
• Do you think about harming yourself?

If the patient (or caregiver) answers "yes" to some or most of the questions, depression may be a concern.

Note: You can also use these questions to assess the caregiver for signs of depression.

Performing the physical exam

QUICK ASSESSMENT

When I need to make a patient assessment in a hurry and still obtain a maximum amount of information, I use the three-step SPADE technique:

First, determine the patient's status (or progress) in relation to his admitting diagnosis.

Next, assess his general status with SPADE: *S*leep, *P*ain, *A*ctivity, *D*iet, *E*limination.

Finally, determine his most important request for assistance: "What's the most important thing you'd like to have help with today?"

This abbreviated assessment will help you in reviewing medical orders with doctors and in planning and implementing nursing care.

WHAT NERVES

When I was in nursing school, I devised this number drawing to help me remember the 12 cranial nerves.

Beneath the drawing, I listed the nerves that correspond with the numbers in the picture. Then I named some of the

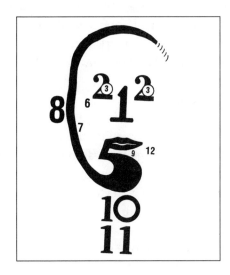

actions or sensations controlled by those nerves. My list
looked like this:

1. Olfactory—smell
2. Optic—vision
3. Oculomotor—iris and eye movements
4. Trochlear—eye movements
5. Trigeminal—upper and lower mouth and teeth, forehead,
anterior half of scalp
6. Abducens—eye movement (lateral)
7. Facial—facial expression
8. Acoustic—hearing, balance
9. Glossopharyngeal—tastebuds on posterior part of
tongue, throat sensations, saliva secretions
10. Vagus—swallowing, vocal cords, goes to abdominal
organs
11. Accessory—head and shoulder movements
12. Hypoglossal—chewing, speaking, swallowing.

The drawing was a handy study aid in school, and it's a
handy reference now.

NERVE TEST KIT

For testing a patient's cranial nerves, I carry a small kit that
contains cotton, safety pins, pennies, keys, peppermint, reflex
hammer, tuning fork, pencil, tongue blade, and an ophthal-
moscope. For convenience, I mark each item with the name
and number of the cranial nerve function it tests.

PINPOINTING PUPIL SIZE

Determining a patient's pupil size is an important part of
neurologic checks. But in recording the size, nurses sometimes use vague terminology that can be open to interpretation. For instance, a pupil that appears "moderate" in size to
one person may appear "dilated" to someone else.

To estimate and record pupil size more accurately, I carry a
chart of pupil sizes on electrocardiograph paper. A pinpoint
pupil is 1 mm—the size of one small square. A moderate-

sized pupil is 5 mm—the size of a large square. A fully dilated pupil is 8 or 9 mm.

LIGHTING UP AT WORK

I keep a small, disposable flashlight (the kind sold for key chains) attached to my stethoscope. I use it for neurologic checks and for looking in the patient's throat. The flashlight is also a good distraction for younger patients. It's inexpensive and comes in various colors.

GETTING A REACTION

Here's a way I can check pupil reactivity without using a penlight. First, I turn on all the lights in the room and ask the patient to look directly at me with both eyes. Then, I cover one of the patient's eyes with my hand, watching for dilation (accommodation) in the other eye. Next, I remove my hand and watch for constriction (direct light reflex) in the eye that was covered. Test the other eye the same way.

QUICK NEUROLOGIC EXAM

Got a few minutes? Sometimes, I must assess a patient's neurologic status that quickly. When time's short, here's how I handle the assessment:
• Evaluate mental status and speech.
• Test cranial nerves II, III, IV, V, VI, and VII for function.
• Assess balance and gait.
• Test wrist and arm extension, foot dorsiflexion, and knee flexion.
• Check sensation in both arms and legs.
• Test biceps, triceps, patellar, and Achilles reflexes.

   Later, when time permits, I do a thorough neurologic assessment.

TWO THINGS AT ONCE

When assessing a patient's motor system and time is short, I inspect the patient's muscles and look for abnormal muscle movement at the same time I test for muscle tone and strength.

HALF ASLEEP
Whenever I rouse a patient from a deep sleep, I make sure the patient is fully awake before I proceed with a neurologic assessment.

PALPATING THE ABDOMEN
Before palpating a patient's abdomen, I ask the patient if any areas are tender. If yes, I palpate those areas last so I don't cause undue stress.

AUSCULTATING BRUITS
From experience, I've learned that auscultating can give unexpected results: a false bruit. Typically, bruits result from arterial lumen narrowing or arterial dilation. But bruits can also come from excessive pressure applied to the stethoscope's bell during auscultation. Too much pressure compresses the artery, creating turbulent blood flow and the false bruit.

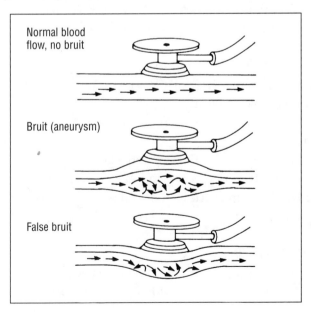

Normal blood flow, no bruit

Bruit (aneurysm)

False bruit

To prevent this, I place the bell lightly on the patient's skin. And if I'm auscultating for a popliteal bruit, I place the patient supine, putting my hand behind the patient's ankle and lifting the leg slightly before placing the bell behind the knee.

MARKING PULSES
When using a Doppler ultrasound stethoscope, I like to mark the patient's peripheral pulses with white liquid correction fluid. Unlike ink, the correction fluid won't dissolve with frequent applications of the gel used to obtain Doppler readings.

TRANSDUCER CLEANING TIP
After using a Doppler transducer to assess pulses, I clean the head of the transducer with a dry gauze pad. Here's a word of caution, however: Don't use alcohol or an abrasive cleaner; either can damage the head and interfere with sound transmission.

X MARKS THE PULSE
Locating pedal and post-tibial pulses can be time-consuming. After I find them, I use a felt-tip pen to mark an X over a palpable pulse and a D over a pulse that's detectable by a Doppler ultrasound stethoscope only.

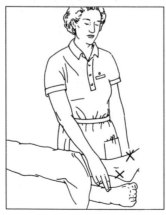

This not only helps the nurse on the next visit, but it also allows us to determine quickly if the pulse has worsened or improved.

CUSHIONING OUT NOISE
If you ever have to take a patient's blood pressure in a noisy place, try my trick: Put a pillow under the patient's antecubital area first. The pillow seems to cut out the distracting noise and allows you to get an accurate blood pressure reading.

CLOSE FIT
Neither too loose, nor too tight. That's my goal when taking a patient's blood pressure. Why? If I wrap the cuff too loosely, I'll get a false-high reading; too tight, I'll get a false low.

REFILL TIME CHECK
To assess my patient's capillary refill time, I press down on the patient's nail bed, release, then say the words "capillary refill."

By the time I've said that, normal color should have returned to the nail.

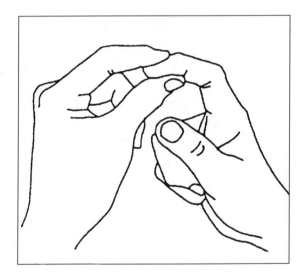

KOROTKOFF'S SOUNDS

If you have trouble hearing Korotkoff's sounds, try this technique, which works for me: Intensify the sounds by increasing vascular pressure below the cuff. Here's how to do it:

Palpate the brachial artery and mark it with an indelible pen. Apply the cuff and ask the patient to raise his arm above his head. Then inflate the cuff about 30 mm Hg above the patient's systolic pressure. Ask the patient to lower his arm until the cuff reaches heart level, deflate the cuff, and take a reading.

Here's an alternative method: Position the patient's arm at heart level and inflate the cuff to 30 mm Hg above the patient's systolic pressure; then ask him to make a fist. Next, ask him to open and close his hand rapidly about 10 times before you begin to deflate the cuff and take the reading.

SITE CHANGES

You probably know that blood pressure varies from upper arm to forearm to leg and from the right side of the body to the left. Fortunately, these variations are predictable.

To determine if a patient's pressure is high or low, all I have to do is remember that blood pressure is usually slightly higher in the forearm than in the upper arm. And systolic leg pressures tend to be about 20 mm Hg higher than systolic arm pressures. Diastolic readings usually remain fairly constant throughout the body.

BLOOD PRESSURE TRENDS

Every time I visit a patient, I take at least two blood pressure readings. Why? A series of blood pressure measurements over time provides more reliable clinical information than a single isolated measurement.

CHEST MOVES

When checking a patient's breathing, I observe the chest closely. Does the patient use the scalene or trapezius muscles for breathing? Are there any supraclavicular retractions? If the answer is yes, the patient may be having trouble inhaling.

MORE CHEST MOVES
Are you having trouble seeing the apical impulse? Here's what I do to make viewing easier: If my patient has large breasts, I move them slightly. If the patient's chest is enlarged from obesity or emphysema, I ask the patient to sit up.

TAKE IT OFF
This may seem obvious, but it's worth a reminder: Don't auscultate a patient's heart through clothing or dressings; both can block sound. And avoid introducing extra noise by keeping the stethoscope tubing off the patient's body or other surfaces.

HEART SOUNDS
Whenever I auscultate a patient's heart, I listen for additional heart sounds. Remember, the rhythm of S_3 resembles that of a galloping horse; its cadence is similar to the word "ken-tuc-ky." And the rhythm of S_4 has the same cadence as the word "ten-nes-see."

VENOUS DISTENTION
Does your patient have right ventricular dysfunction? Then look for jugular venous distention when assessing the patient.

STEADY VISION
It's a natural reaction: If you approach a patient with a bright light, the patient will look away. To prevent such reactions, I explain what's about to happen beforehand. And during an ophthalmoscopic examination, I also place my hand on the patient's shoulder as a reminder not to move, even though I'll be getting extremely close.

STRENGTH TEST TECHNIQUE

Here's how I quickly check the strength of a patient's handgrip: First, I roll up a blood pressure cuff, pump it up slightly, and ask the patient to squeeze it while I measure the millimeters of mercury. Then I do the same thing with the patient's other hand. The reading for the dominant hand may be higher by 10 to 20 mm Hg. This technique can help detect slight neurologic changes, saving the patient from potential problems.

STRENGTH TEST SAFETY TIP

Caution's always appropriate, and it certainly applies when I'm testing a patient's strength. Instead of extending my entire hand for the patient to squeeze, I extend only two or three fingers; an overzealous patient may unintentionally squeeze hard enough to hurt.

SKIN BREAKDOWN: MIRROR IMAGE

When I'm caring for a patient who can't turn over—I use a small mirror to check the heels for skin breakdown. Just lift the patient's leg slightly, and place the mirror under the heel; then assess the image.

KEEPING A STETHOSCOPE STERILE

Preventing cross-contamination is very important. So before I auscultate a patient's chest and abdomen, I place a rubber glove over my stethoscope's diaphragm. I can still hear heart, breath, and bowel sounds, as well as the patient's pulse when I take a blood pressure reading—yet the diaphragm won't be contaminated with body fluids draining from a patient's wounds. When I'm finished, I dispose of the glove and wipe the diaphragm with an alcohol pad to help prevent cross-contamination.

MACULE OR PAPULE?

Here's a quick and easy way to determine whether a lesion is a macule or a papule: In low light, shine a penlight or flashlight at a right angle to the lesion. If the light casts a shadow, the lesion is a papule. Macules are flat and won't produce a shadow.

LEFT OR RIGHT?

My patient has suffered a stroke; I'm certain of that. But which side? To help identify whether it's a left- or right-sided cerebrovascular accident (CVA), I concentrate on these assessment findings:

• Left-sided CVA: right-sided (opposite side) paralysis, possible speech and language deficits, slow and cautious behavior, right-left disorientation, vision changes, fear, and emotional instability.

• Right-sided CVA: left-sided (opposite side) paralysis, euphoria, tendency to be easily distracted, impulsive behavior, vision changes, and indifference or denial related to the episode.

THE FIVE Ps

I check the five Ps to determine my patient's peripheral vascular circulation:

1. Pain
2. Pallor
3. Paresthesia
4. Pulselessness
5. Paralysis

If my patient has all five signs, I can anticipate that he has an acute arterial occlusion and will need emergency treatment.

ASTHMA AND WHEEZING

If you're unable to auscultate wheezing during an asthma attack, here's why: When a patient experiences severe bronchospasm, there isn't enough air movement available to create the turbulence that causes wheezing. So breath sounds may be greatly reduced, but without adventitious sounds. When this happens, the patient is in acute hypoventilation—an emergency situation.

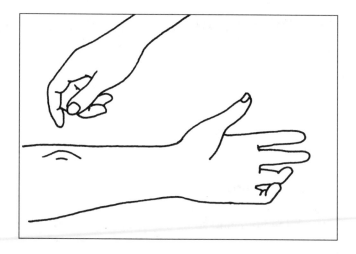

SKIN PICK-UP TEST

Here's an easy way to assess skin turgor, or resiliency, in an adult: Pick up a fold of skin over the sternum or arm. Then release the fold. Normally, the skin will return immediately to its previous position. With decreased turgor, the fold will remain for up to 30 seconds.

SKIN COLOR DIFFERENCES

Cyanosis can be difficult to detect in dark-skinned patients. Here's what you'll need to look for: a bluish discoloration of the mucous membranes in the mouth and under the tongue, and on the inner eyelids.

THE SPIN ON ELDERLY SKIN

To accurately assess skin turgor in an elderly patient, try squeezing the skin of the sternum or forehead, instead of using the forearm. In an elderly patient, the skin of the forearm tends to be flaccid so using the site to assess skin turgor wouldn't give you an accurate evaluation of the patient's hydration.

Obtaining accurate measurements

MAPPING SKIN CONDITION

Even careful documentation of a patient's skin condition
doesn't always tell the story as clearly as possible. That's the
reason I include a "Rule of Nines" form—minus the numbers—with my written notes in the nursing care plan. Here's
what I do:

I indicate all skin abnormalities on the anatomic form by
marking the appropriate areas with red ink. I also write a
brief description of the abnormality, including size, appear-
ance, type of wound, and so forth. This gives a picture that's
truly worth a thousand words.

MEASURING LEG PAIN: STEP-BY-STEP

As you know, a patient with arterial peripheral vascular disease usually experiences leg pain that intensifies with walking.
What you don't know is exactly how far that patient can walk
without such pain. Vague descriptions, such as "only a short
distance," "not too far," or "from my house to the street corner" don't allow you to judge the severity of his disease.

For a more accurate assessment, have him count the number of steps he takes before he feels pain. This gives you
objective data that you can use to measure the patient's
progress.

MORE THAN HEMS

A 6" (15-cm) hem gauge can do more than just measure
hems; it can also measure the size of lacerations or contu-
sions and the amount of bleeding or drainage on surgical
dressings and casts.

I carry the gauge with me throughout the day—it takes up
no more room in my bag or pocket than a pen or bandage
scissors.

A MEASURING DEVICE YOU CAN'T MISPLACE

Measuring devices, such as rulers and tapes, present the same problem as pens and pencils: They're easy to lose. But here's a substitute that's simple to use, water resistant, and portable. Best of all, it never gets lost, and it's always at hand. The device: your hand. In order to use it accurately, measure parts, such as the nail bed of your little finger and the first joint to the tip of your index finger; then memorize the measurements.

FLUID STATUS

My patient's weight varied by almost 6 pounds (2.7 kg) on 3 days over 2 weeks. I didn't notice any pattern to the variations at first, until I quizzed the patient and caregiver. Seems that on some mornings the patient stepped on the scale in his pajamas and bare feet, before breakfast; other times, the patient got on the scale fully dressed, including shoes, after eating breakfast.

The incident served as a reminder to me that patients and their families know little about assessing fluid status. Now, I remember to tell them that weight must be taken at the same time every day, using the same scale, wearing the same type of clothing.

A significant weight gain or loss within 24 to 48 hours indicates a change in fluid status, not in body mass. Loss can be from perspiration and breathing, as well as from vomiting, diarrhea, fever, and wound drainage. Weight gain can result from fluid overload, excessive salt intake or overadministering I.V. fluids.

PITTING EDEMA

Checking one of my patients for edema is quick when I do it this way: First, I press firmly for 5 to 10 seconds over a bony area, such as the subcutaneous part of the tibia, fibula, sacrum, or sternum. Then I remove my finger and note the depth and duration of the depression (or pit).

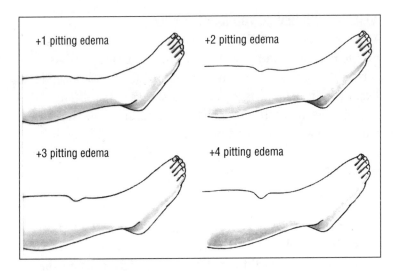

+1 pitting edema

+2 pitting edema

+3 pitting edema

+4 pitting edema

I document my observation on a scale from +1 (brief and barely detectable) to +4 (a persistent pit as deep as 1" [2.5 cm]).

HOW DEEP A WOUND?

This is the best way to measure the depth of a wound:

• Saturate the tip of a sterile, flexible cotton-tipped applicator with normal saline solution, and insert the applicator into the deepest part of the wound.

• Grasp the applicator with your thumb and forefinger at skin level, and withdraw it without changing your finger position.

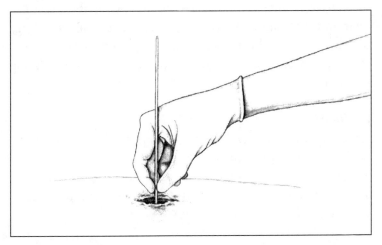

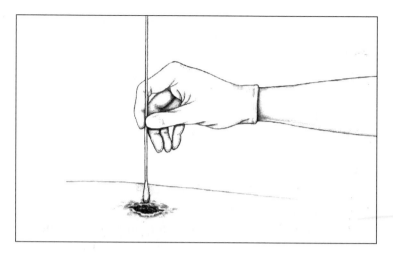

• Align the applicator with a ruler, and measure from the applicator's tip to your fingers.
• Record the wound depth in centimeters on a tracing of the wound.

Assessing pain

WHERE DOES IT HURT?

When a patient complains of pain, I ask questions: How bad is it? Where is it located? Is the pain dull? Sharp? Constant? And I watch the patient's face, looking for wincing or a tense expression. I also carry a photocopy of a body chart, which I've laminated, so the patient can show me exactly where it hurts.

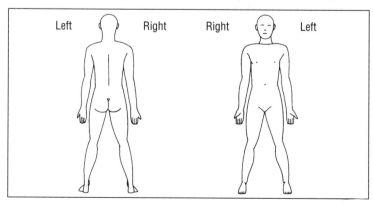

Another help in assessing pain: To encourage the patient to participate in monitoring his pain, I make a large photocopy of the human body and leave it in his home. If the patient has intermittent pain, he can mark the chart when I'm not there.

RATING PAIN

Question: "How bad is your pain?"
Answer: "Real bad . . . I guess."

Sound familiar? Unfortunately, most patients have difficulty describing their pain accurately. To help my patients (and me) get a handle on their level of pain, I use a pain assessment scale on which I ask the patient to mark the spot that corresponds to the degree of pain. Remember to assess for each source of pain if there's more than one.

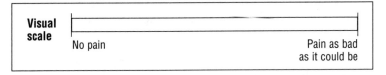

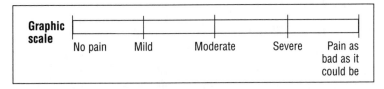

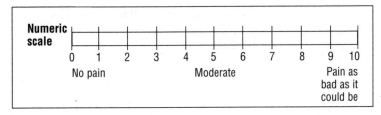

3

The Adult Patient

Contents

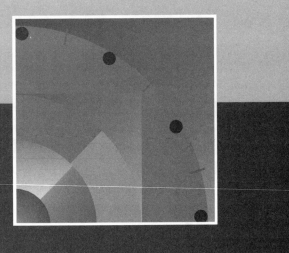

Contributors

The following nurses and health care providers
contributed tips and timesavers for this chapter:

Ann Barrow, RN, MSN, CCRN

Patricia Kardish Fischer, RN, BSN

Collette Bishop Hendler, RN, CCRN

Judith Schilling McCann, RN, MSN

Mary Beth Morrell, RN, CCRN

Lori Neri, RN, MSN, CCRN

Terry Poiesz, RT(T), BS

Patricia Dwyer Schull, RN, MSN

Beverly Ann Tscheschlog, RN

Skin care

OVERCOMING WOUND ODORS

Patients experience many stressors when recovering from surgery. For many patients under my care, embarrassing odors emanating from a healing wound are a serious problem. Here are two techniques to overcome persistent wound odor:

• Irrigate the wound with Dakin's solution, dress it with Dakin's saturated gauze, and cover it with an absorbent secondary dressing, such as foam or extra-absorbent surgical dressing.

• Change the dressing more often and use an odor-absorbing product, such as Bard Absorption Dressing.

SOOTHING AN ITCH

If one of my patients complains of vulvovaginal itching, I suggest she do the following:

• Take daily showers and wash between showers with soap and water.

• Avoid tub baths.

• Wear white cotton underwear and change it daily.

• Avoid using feminine hygiene deodorant products.

• Use white, unscented toilet tissue.

• Wipe the perineal area from front to back.

ONE GOOD TURN DESERVES ANOTHER

Every day patients susceptible to pressure ulcers need to be turned and turned again. To help the family remember when

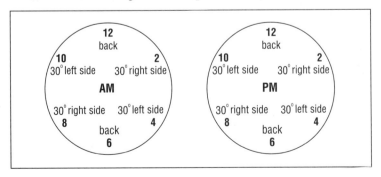

to turn the patient, I suggest they use a "turn clock"— a hand-drawn clock with turning times and patient positions.

RELIEVING COLD SORES

Inconvenient, embarrassing, and painful, all describe the common cold sore, for which there is no cure. But some relief is possible. Here's what I suggest my patients do:
• Apply cool compresses.
• Take aspirin or other pain medication as directed on the package.
• Avoid acidic foods and beverages, such as grapefruit juice, that irritate the sore.
• Use an over-the-counter cold sore remedy.
• Call their doctor if the cold sore does not heal in 10 days.

Respiratory care

COPD: PLANNING THE PATIENT'S PACE

A simple fact of life for patients with chronic obstructive pulmonary disease (COPD): Activities that you and I do easily, like brushing our teeth and combing our hair, can be exhausting. That's why I focus on helping my patients use their energy wisely.

"Plan your day to conserve energy," I tell them, suggesting that they space personal care activities (shaving, washing, shampooing) over the course of the day. Also, I teach them to exhale when they're exerting energy for activities such as climbing stairs or lifting a package. Too often, people hold their breath during exertion. Muscles, however, need a continual supply of fresh oxygen.

VENTILATION TO GO

Don't let a home ventilator keep an otherwise mobile patient homebound. Instead, encourage the patient to get about. Many ventilators are small enough to be portable and will run on a 12-volt external or internal battery. The external battery is similar to a car battery and will last about 10 hours; the internal battery will run for 1 to 2 hours.

HOME VENTILATOR THERAPY THOUGHTS

In my home health practice, I am caring for more and more patients who are receiving ventilator therapy. Here are six basic rules I devised for ensuring safe home ventilator therapy:
• Become familiar with the ventilator.
• Check the settings frequently to make sure they are correct.
• Keep the ventilator plugged in at all times to avoid draining the battery.
• Know how to switch to the backup battery, and be sure that the patient and caregiver know as well.
• Replace the disposable ventilator tubing weekly.
• Be aware that the manufacturer usually changes ventilator units approximately every 6 months.

PREVENTING OXYGEN OVERLOAD

When caring for a patient on a home ventilator, I usually adjust ventilator settings to administer extra oxygen right before suctioning. One thing that's absolutely crucial: Remember to return the FIO_2 to the ordered setting. A high concentration of oxygen for a short time is okay; too much for a long time may damage the patient's lung tissue.

ACCURATE ABGs

When caring for a home ventilator patient, making changes to ventilator settings and performing suctioning may affect the patient's arterial blood gas (ABG) levels. After I make adjustments or suction the patient's airway, I always wait at least 30 minutes before taking an ABG sample.

READY FOR WEANING?

When I anticipate that a patient is going to be weaned from home ventilator therapy, I am always careful to monitor the patient's inspiratory pressure. A reading below -20 cm H_2O suggests that the patient is not ready for weaning.

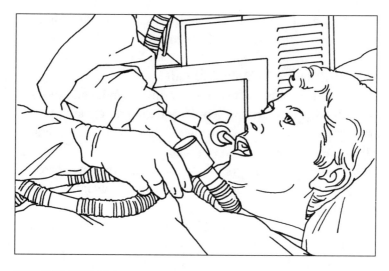

REFLEX RESPONSE

When I worked with a tracheostomy patient for the first time, here is something that surprised me: When I asked the patient to take a deep breath, he opened his mouth. I found out later that this is a common reflex action in tracheostomy patients.

Nutrition

EASY TO SWALLOW

Here are two techniques that may help a patient who has difficulty swallowing:

• Have the patient sit upright with his head tilted forward.
• For the patient who has difficulty swallowing liquids, try offering semi-frozen or thicker liquids; for example, rather than serving plain milk, mix it into a milkshake.

SWEET SUBSTITUTIONS

During my home visits to diabetic patients, I am often asked what is an appropriate remedy for a hypoglycemic attack. Many patients have been told to mix sugar into a glass of orange juice. Here's what I tell them:

• Adding packets of sugar to orange juice is rarely necessary.
• Any of the following can be used to bolster blood sugar levels: half-cup of soft drink (with real sugar), half-cup of orange juice, or 1 cup of low-fat milk.
• Swallowing glucose tablets or sucking on hard candy may also alleviate hypoglycemic episodes.

HUNGRY FOR YELLOW?

Helping a patient who has little appetite get adequate nutrition is one of the most difficult challenges of home care nursing. Believe it or not, I encourage the patient and families to create colorful surroundings to stimulate the appetite. Studies suggest that yellow, red, and orange stimulate the appetite, whereas blue, green, and dark colors depress the appetite. That's why I recommend using a colorful tablecloth, placemat, and napkin.

THE 10-SECOND CANCER RISK-REDUCING DIET

Many of my patients have learned about the relationship between cancer and diet from television shows or from magazine articles. Occasionally, they will ask me for advice on this topic. I use the following simple guidelines to encourage dietary changes to reduce cancer risks:
• Eat more high fiber foods, such as fruits, vegetables, and whole grain cereals.
• Include dark green and deep yellow fruits and vegetables rich in vitamin C in your diet daily.
• Eat cabbage, broccoli, Brussels sprouts, kohlrabi, and cauliflower often.
• Consume less salt-cured, smoked, and nitrate-cured foods.
• Reduce total fat intake from animal sources and fats and oils.
• Lose weight (if obese).
• Drink alcohol in moderation.

DO-IT-YOURSELF FLUID REPLACEMENT

I care for several homebound patients who may need ready access to rehydration solution. I make a point of teaching

these patients how to mix their own fluid-and-electrolyte replacement solution, if it's ever necessary. Here are two recipes:
• Mix 8 ounces apple, apricot, or orange juice (the patient can substitute another juice, but it must have lots of potassium) with a pinch of table salt and ½ teaspoon corn syrup or honey.
• Mix 8 ounces water with ¼ teaspoon baking soda. *Caution:* If you suspect the patient's water source isn't pure, use boiled, bottled, or carbonated water.

RULES FOR REDUCING REFLUX
Several patients under my care complain of reflux associated with hiatal hernia. I recommend they do the following to reduce occurrences of reflux:
• Eat small, frequent meals.
• Eat slowly and sit up while eating.
• Eat small evening meals at least 3 hours before bedtime.
• Avoid acidic juices, caffeinated and carbonated beverages, raw fruits, highly seasoned foods, and foods high in fat.
• Keep weight within normal range.

Mobility, exercise, and rest

HOOKED ON CROCHET
Once I was caring for an elderly woman who loved to crochet, but arthritis had made holding a crochet hook painful

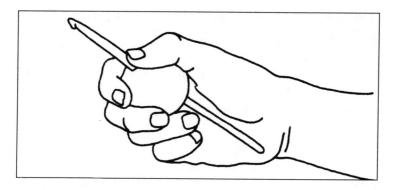

and difficult. I did not want to see her abandon a hobby she loved, so I devised an easy-to-make handgrip for her crochet hook. I simply poke the hooks through a small Styrofoam ball. Then I let the patient slide the ball to a position on the hook where she can grip it comfortably and move it efficiently. The handgrip adapts nicely to pens and pencils, too.

You'll need to experiment with different-sized Styrofoam balls until you find the one that gives your patient the most comfortable grip.

COMFORT FOR THE BEDRIDDEN

Occasionally, I've succeeded in increasing a bedridden patient's comfort by raising the head of the bed. Here are two ways to do it (you may need the help of a colleague or family member):
• Wedge a bean bag chair between the bed's mattress and box spring to raise the head of the mattress about 30 degrees.
• Place a few boards or books under the legs at the head of the bed.

CANE CARE

Here's a technique I devised for making life a little easier for my patients who use a cane:

Attach a small piece of Velcro to the handle of the patient's cane and attach a matching piece wherever the patient usually props the cane; for example, the patient's belt, a counter, or a chair. Instruct the patient to hang the cane from the Velcro when he isn't using it. This way, the cane will stay upright and is less likely to fall on the floor and create a safety hazard.

THE BEST CAST REST

I picked up this strategy for helping a patient with a cast courtesy of a home care nursing colleague:

Teach the patient to use a crutch to prop up the casted leg, as shown on page 42. After the patient sits down, he should adjust the crutch to the shortest position; then place it

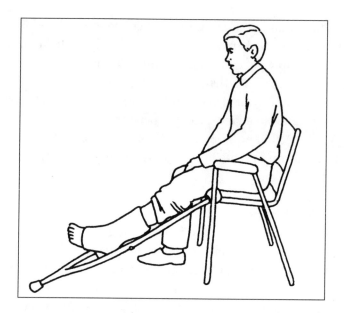

between his chair and thigh, with the hand grip pointing away from him. He can place his casted leg over the crutch so his ankle is supported by the hand grip and his foot rests below the grip.

Because the crutch goes wherever the patient goes, the patient will always be able to elevate and steady the leg while sitting.

STOCKING STORY

Home care patients who must put on antiembolism stockings may experience difficulty or frustration. Here is a tip I offer my patients to make this task easier:

Use stockings with a toe window. Slip a plastic bag over the foot and pull the stocking up over the bag. Once the toes are exposed, pull the plastic bag off through the toe window of the stocking.

RELAXATION TECHNIQUES

Before using techniques that require your patient to stretch his muscles, try relaxing your patient's muscles with vibration (such as is used in chest physiotherapy) or by applying pressure to the area. Consider using such techniques in any situation in which you want to help relax the muscles; doing so helps to improve the patient's ability to stretch without injury.

RELIEF FOR SORE MUSCLES

Have a patient who's bothered by sore muscles; for example, a patient who's been lying in bed too long? Try kneading the muscle to provide relief. Kneading, also called petrissage, is a technique that uses an alternating grasping and compressing motion. It helps bring about relief from chronic pain, especially from sore muscles and underlying joint problems. Be sure to monitor for underlying joint problems first.

ICE ADVICE

If your patient uses an ice pack to relieve pain, remind him not to use it for longer than 30 minutes at a time. Prolonged use can result in frostbite.

FALL NO MORE

Most falls happen in the patient's home. Falls are especially dangerous for patients who have osteoporosis. To reduce the risks, I make a point of providing patients and family members with the following list of tips:
• Eliminate throw, or scatter, rugs.
• Arrange furniture so it's not an obstacle.
• Eliminate clutter.
• Keep rooms well lit.
• Install grab bars in the bathroom.
    I also suggest that women avoid wearing high-heeled shoes; low-heeled shoes give better support.

SWEET DREAMS

Many of my patients complain of not being able to sleep at night. Here's a quick list of patient teaching tips for getting a

good night's sleep that I like to share:
• Go to bed at the same time each night; awake at the same time each day.
• Exercise regularly.
• Avoid eating large meals before going to bed.
• Don't drink caffeine or alcohol before going to bed.
• Stay away from over-the-counter sleep aids.
• Practice deep breathing and relaxation techniques.
• Drink a glass of warm milk before going to bed.

NECK STRAIN STOPPER

Returning home from the hospital after a thyroidectomy, one of my patients complained of severe neck strain and pain from the incision. To help the patient relieve the stress on her neck, I instructed her to place her hands behind her neck for support whenever she wanted to turn her head. It also proved helpful for her to support her head with a pillow and put her hands together behind her neck when rising to a sitting position in bed.

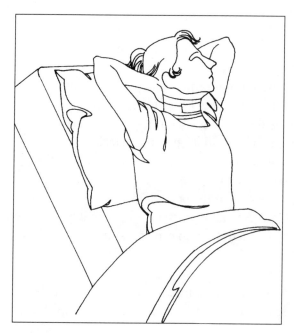

ENERGY SAVERS

I make regular visits to a patient with congestive heart failure who tires very easily. Just buttoning a shirt is exhausting for this patient. These suggestions have helped him conserve much-needed energy:
• Use dressing aids, such as a long-handled shoehorn or zipper pull.
• Wear mittens; they're easier to pull on than gloves.
• Use household aids, such as a hand-held shower nozzle and grab bars.
• Sit down as much as possible; for example, sit when buttoning a jacket, when showering, when putting on a belt.

Infection control

AIDS LAUNDRY LIST

I work for an agency that provides care for AIDS patients, and we recommend that all nurses and caregivers take extra precautions when handling an AIDS patient's laundry. Here's a list of our recommendations:
• Wear gloves when handling any soiled clothing or linens.
• Launder the patient's items separately from other people's.
• Wash towels and washcloths immediately after the patient uses them.
• Use hot water, detergent, and bleach, and use the high setting on the dryer.

What if the caregiver can't get to the laundry for a day or two? The caregiver should seal the soiled laundry in a heavy-duty, double plastic bag until the wash can be done.

SHARP ABOUT SHARPS

Working with AIDS patients has taught me to be cautious when disposing of sharps. Now, I always place them in an impervious container, such as a coffee can, heavy-duty plastic detergent bottle, or glass jar. I always check to make sure the container has a lid.

GLOVE GUIDELINES

I work for an agency where the staff is very safety-minded. If we must perform several procedures on the same patient, we wear fresh gloves with each procedure. This is to ensure protection if the gloves sustain tiny holes or rips.

MASK MATTERS

I enjoy sharing information I learn from colleagues and reading. Here's something I learned recently: If you have to wear a face mask (for example, because of barrier precautions) keep in mind it may become ineffective when moist. So, when you are required to wear a mask, keep conversation minimal (to keep the mask dry) and have several backup masks handy (in case it gets wet).

ADDING TO A STERILE FIELD

When you perform home health care procedures that must be sterile, remember the following: Never reach across the sterile field when adding items to the field. Instead, go around to the other side and let the new items drop onto the sterile field (rather than reaching over). Take care that the sterile item never touches an unsterile surface.

Eyes and ears

TROUBLESHOOTING HEARING AIDS

Does your patient's hearing aid whistle and squeal? If so, this is what I would do: Have the patient take out the earmold and then reinsert it, turn down the volume, and check the connection between the earmold and the receiver. If you still can't find the source of the problem, advise the patient to have the hearing aid taken in for repairs.

EYE PROTECTION POINTERS

Most of my patients are fairly well informed about protecting their skin from the harmful effects of the sun. But many fail to realize that they must also protect their eyes. So when I discuss sun protection measures, I also stress the importance of wearing sunglasses that have been treated to block UVA and UVB rays. Studies indicate that ultraviolet radiation from the sun penetrates the eye's clear lens and contributes to premature cataracts.

CLEAR THE EARS

I remember one home visit when family members were very anxious and upset. The day before, their mother had experienced a sudden loss of hearing. The condition turned out to have a simple explanation: it resulted from an accumulation of cerumen, the natural substance created by oil glands in the ear canal.

Communication

SILENT NO MORE

Here are some simple ways to communicate with a patient who's lost the ability to speak.

• Use a magic slate if the patient can write.

• Use an alphabet board, magnetic alphabet letters, or blocks if the patient can't write.

• Phrase questions so they require only "yes" or "no" answers; the patient need write or pick up only a "y" for "yes" or an "n" for "no."

EMERGENCY TAPES

For the patient who can't speak, wise use of a tape recorder can save the day, literally. Have someone tape-record several emergency phone messages on the patient's behalf that can be played over the phone to the local fire company, police department, and ambulance service. Also, tape a message for the patient's doctor. These messages increase the patient's level of independence and foster confidence in his ability to get help when necessary.

4

The Geriatric Patient

Contents

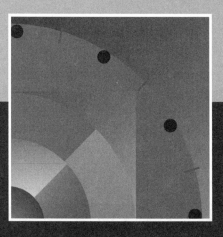

Contributors

The following nurses provided tips and timesavers for this chapter:

Nancy J. Augustine, RN

Pam Barton, RN

Jane Marie Brown, RN

Debora J. Burke, RN

Maxine Chisholm, MSN, GNP

Angelina Elkin, RN

B. Felker, RN

Melissa Gilliland, RN

Margaret Guilfoyle, RN

Linda Jeronovitz, RN

J. Kelly, LPN

Valrie Loftes, LPN

Barbara Malcomb, RN, PHN

Tina Marks, RN, MS

Sandra McIntosh, LPN

Leah McNulty, RN, BSN

Vicki L. Miller, LPN

Jane Mooney, CNA-CMT

Jan M. Moroni, RN, BSN

Joyce Nelson, RN, BSN

Ruth L. Nermal, RN

Arlene Orhon Jech, RN

Kay Preshlock, RN, BS

Debbie Sanders, RN

Karen Seifert, RN

Carol Taylor, RN, MSN

Evelyn R. White, RN

Assistive devices

BIG NUMBERS

For my elderly home health care patients who can't see the small numbers on their stoves and microwaves, I put brightly colored stickers above the numbers they use most. This way they can more easily recognize the numbers and temperatures, preventing them from burning themselves and starting fires.

SPECIAL SPOONS

To feed an elderly patient, try using a small, plastic-coated spoon (the kind used for babies). The spoon holds a more manageable portion that's easier to swallow. Plus, the soft coating is less irritating to sensitive gums.

CUP CONTROL

Even if he's using a straw, a patient may have trouble drinking from a cup. A training cup may solve the problem. These cups have handles on both sides and a lid on top, so the patient can drink by himself and still have some control. And if he drops it, he won't make much of a mess.

CUP OF ENCOURAGEMENT

An elderly patient had trouble drinking out of a regular glass and refused to drink through a straw. So I asked his family to buy a plastic cup with a sipper lid. Because the patient was

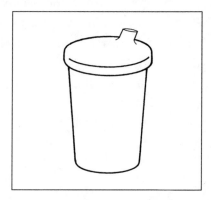

able to use this cup without spills, he could drink the required amount of fluid each day.

TEAMWORK

One of my elderly home care patients is a big man who's too debilitated to pull himself up in bed. His wife, a small woman, isn't strong enough to pull him up either. With a little ingenuity and teamwork, though, they discovered a way to move him.

They twisted a flat bed sheet into a rope and placed it across the bed, under the patient's shoulders. They brought the ends of the sheet under his armpits, over his shoulders, and over the head of the bed. Then the wife grips each end and, with the patient pushing with his feet, she can pull him up in bed.

Improvising procedures and equipment

MANICURE THERAPY

Ever try conducting a manicure session for elderly patients? You'll be surprised how a simple activity like this can generate fun and interest. As an added benefit, manicuring offers an opportunity to encourage finger movement.

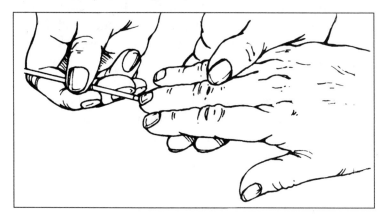

BRUSH UP ON FUN

Some elderly patients with limited mobility in their hands, such as those who have arthritis or paralysis, may be missing out on some fun because they can't hold playing cards or magazines. To help them participate in such activities, give them a scrub brush. With the bristle end up, the brush can hold cards, pictures, and even light magazines.

CUSTOM GOWN: QUICK CUT

Here's an easy way for a family member to make a gown for a home health care patient: Have the family member cut a cotton nightgown up the back and hem the edges so that they don't fray. The result is a gown that works great for a bedridden patient, especially if he's incontinent.

ELBOW PROTECTORS

An elderly home care patient wanted some elbow protectors. I didn't have any with me, so I suggested she make them herself.

I told her to cut the tops and toes off an old pair of socks. She could then place a sanitary pad (with an adhesive strip) inside each sock, lengthwise over the heel. This makes a pair of comfortable, inexpensive elbow (or heel) protectors.

IMPROVISING AN ENEMA

As a home health care nurse, I sometimes have to improvise procedures. I once used the following technique to administer an enema to an elderly patient who didn't have the necessary supplies.

I positioned the patient on a rubber pad on her left side with her right knee drawn up to her chest. Then I lubricated about 6" (15 cm) of the end of a sterile #16 French catheter with K-Y jelly and inserted the catheter slowly and gently into the patient's rectum.

Next, I attached a 60-ml irrigating syringe filled with the enema solution to the end of the catheter. By raising or lowering the syringe, I could control the flow of water into the rectum.

SUBSTITUTE STRAPS

One of my elderly home care patients had an indwelling urinary catheter with a leg bag. The straps on the bag dug into his skin, causing irritation. In looking for substitute straps for the bag, I noticed the strap on a Depend adult disposable undergarment. This strap is wide and stretchy, and it has two buttons on each end. I wrapped the strap around the patient's leg and attached the leg bag to the buttons. The strap stays in place and doesn't harm the patient's skin.

TRACKING FLUID FLOW

To help my fluid-restricted home health care patient keep track of his fluid intake, I tell him to put an empty quart container in the kitchen each morning. (If your patient is allowed a different amount of fluid, mark the container accordingly or use one of a different size.) Every time he takes a drink, he pours an equal amount of fluid into the container. When the container is full, he knows he's had his limit.

COLOR CODING

An elderly blind woman who lives alone recently told me how she coordinates the colors in her wardrobe: She uses safety pins to code the clothing by color. For instance, one pin placed on a garment in a vertical position indicates that the garment is white. Two vertical pins indicate that the garment is blue. Pins placed horizontally indicate other colors.

The coding system helps the woman retain her independence because it allows her to dress properly without assistance.

GERIATRICKS

Collecting a urine specimen from an elderly woman patient when you can't get an order for an indwelling or straight catheter can be difficult. So try using a pediatric urine bag. Tape the bag over the patient's perineum. It holds about 50 to 60 ml of urine—sufficient for most tests.

COLLECTION GLOVE

Here's how we can collect urine specimens from incontinent male patients: We turn an examining glove inside out and place it over the patient's penis. After taping the glove in place, we put a disposable adult incontinence pad on him.

Using a glove is less expensive than using a catheter, and turning it inside out prevents powder from getting in the specimen. If the glove overflows, the incontinence pad prevents leakage.

TOURNIQUET SUBSTITUTE

It's never a good idea to use a tourniquet to dilate an elderly patient's veins before venipuncture. His veins may look healthy but may actually be quite fragile; a tourniquet can cause a hematoma when the needle pierces the vein.

Instead, ask the patient to hang his arm at his side for a few minutes while he opens and closes his fist. Then, lightly tap the area around the vein to dilate it. If you must use a tourniquet, use only light pressure.

SPEAK SLOWLY

In my home care visits, I encounter many elderly patients with progressive hearing loss. Here are some rules I've learned to enhance communication:
• Speak slowly and keep your voice pitch normal.
• Keep your hands away from your face when you speak.
• Ask the patient to turn off the television or radio before you speak. Alternatively, find another, quieter place to talk.

• Wait quietly for the patient to answer your questions.
• Keep explanations brief and be sure the patient understands you before you go on to another topic.

Medication administration

QUICK CRUSH
I work primarily with geriatric patients, and I have to crush a lot of medications. I've found a quick, sanitary way to do that. I put the tablet in a paper cup and place an empty cup inside the first, on top of the tablet. Then I pound a heavy-handled knife or meat tenderizer mallet into the top cup. This easily crushes the tablet, and the pieces are neatly contained in one cup.

DOSAGE MARKERS
Elderly diabetic patients who give themselves insulin some-times have trouble reading the unit markings on the syringe. To prevent a dosage error, use a marking pen or colored nail polish to mark the correct number of units on each syringe.

COOL DROPS
Because elderly patients have difficulty sensing drops in the eye, I suggest they chill the medication. Cold drops will be easier to feel when administered.

EASY READING
Many of the elderly patients under my care have difficulty reading labels on prescription bottles. If you encounter this problem, consider suggesting that the patient purchase a magnifying glass. Also check with the patient's pharmacy to see if it provides large-print labels. If it does, request that the pharmacy use these labels for every prescription filled by the patient.

Skin care

PROTECTIVE SLEEVE FOR FRAGILE SKIN

Here's an inexpensive way to protect an elderly patient's fragile skin:

Cut a piece of orthopedic stockinette that's long enough to cover the patient's arm from the hand to the elbow. Slip the stockinette over his arm; then cut a small hole to slide his thumb through (this will hold the stockinette in place).

Now if he bumps his arm, his skin will be less likely to tear. Just remember to remove the stockinette as needed for skin care and assessment.

ON GUARD

The skin of elderly patients can be very frail. I find that maintaining skin integrity in geriatric patients is a constant challenge. Here is one technique I believe is helpful:

Place shin guards over the patient's arms and legs to minimize skin tears. The cloth-covered foam guards provide a protective barrier against hard surfaces. Also, the pads help reduce hypothermia by keeping the extremities warm.

COMFORTING CUSHION

I'd like to share some techniques nurses in my agency use to prevent skin breakdown in elderly patients:
• We cushion the patient's bony prominences with sanitary pads when he is sitting down.
• For a patient with arm slings, we wrap a long sanitary pad in a disposable washcloth and place it under the strap around the patient's neck.

FOOT CARE FOR THE ELDERLY

If an elderly patient has toe contractures, you might have difficulty giving him proper foot care. Here's what I do to solve the problem:

I clean his toes with a disposable, sponge-tipped toothbrush. A toothbrush easily fits between the toes without having to spread them apart. I dry the skin after cleaning and apply powder as ordered.

This procedure works well, and it's comfortable for the patient.

REDUCING SKIN TEARS
Before starting an I.V. infusion on an elderly patient, we wrap a 1" × 6" (2.5 × 15 cm) piece of foam around his arm. (We've found that foam packaged in some I.V. catheter sets is the right size.) We tape the foam to the patient's arm so only 1" of tape at both ends touches the skin. Then we can tape the I.V. tubing to the foam. When we remove the tape on the tubing, we don't tear sensitive skin.

Safety measures

WRIST RESTRAINT REPLACEMENT
To prevent an elderly patient from pulling out his feeding tube or catheter without using wrist restraints, which restrict mobility, try this technique.

With the patient's fingers extended, wrap a piece of soft cloth around each hand. Then take two small inflatable tubes (the kind used on children's arms for swimming) and slide them onto the patient's hands. This prevents the patient from being able to manipulate his fingers. As a bonus, the tubes can help prevent contractures by maintaining good hand position.

STAYING AFLOAT
When elderly patients can't tolerate showers, try bathing them on an inflatable air mattress in the bathtub. They'll be more comfortable, especially if they have pressure ulcers or bony prominences. Family caregivers find that this technique is helpful for them, too.

SECRETS OF STAIR SAFETY

Falling is always a risk for an elderly person, especially if he lives in a house with lots of stairs. Here are a few tips that family members can use to help make his home safer:

• Paint the first and last steps on the stairs using a color that's different from the room. The paint will make the steps stand out and easier to see.

• If the stairs have a banister, place a knob on the banister at the first and last steps to serve as a signal.

• Outside stairs can become slick when wet. Before painting the steps, add sand to the paint. When the paint dries, you'll have a rough surface that should prevent slipping.

SAFETY ALARM

Here's a safety tip for elderly patients who use a walker, especially those who live alone in apartment buildings: Tie a wall-mount-style fire alarm onto the walker, with the testing button facing the patient. Alert his neighbors that you're doing this. Then if the patient falls, he can press the button, and they'll come to his aid.

Patient teaching

TEACHING SELF-CATHETERIZATION

Our visiting nurse agency has many patients over age 65. Teaching them self-catheterization can be a challenge. Here's what we do.

We tell the patient to attach the red rubber end of the catheter directly to a leg bag before inserting the catheter into his urethra. After catheter insertion, the urine flows into the leg bag. So the patient doesn't have to worry about aiming the catheter end into a receptacle.

This method is especially helpful if the patient has poor mobility or coordination or if he can only use one hand adequately. If he has poor eyesight or hearing, you can tell him to feel the catheter to sense the warmth as the urine begins to flow.

ELDER EDUCATION

In a course on aging, I learned some tips that might be helpful to other nurses working with geriatric patients.

For example, patients who have poor eyesight may have trouble reading your patient education handouts if you use blue paper. Use nonglare, yellow paper instead. Or if yellow paper isn't available, use a yellow highlighter to emphasize important points. If possible, have your printed materials enlarged so the letters, numbers, and words are easier to read.

Finally, because some of your patients may have a problem with short-term memory, frequently review and reinforce the points in your lesson.

"WHAT IF" TEACHING TECHNIQUE

I find that older patients tend to learn best when you appeal to their knowledge and experience rather than lecture them. That's why I try to incorporate a problem-solving approach into my teaching plans. For example, I use "what if" scenarios to reinforce important points. Here are some sample questions I might ask after going over a topic:

• What if you need two prescriptions but have money for only one?

• What preparations can you make to help control your bladder and bowels before going on a day-long trip?

• What would you do if you were home alone and fell?

Get to know your patients and make teaching something you do *with* them, not *to* them.

5

The Pediatric Patient

Contents

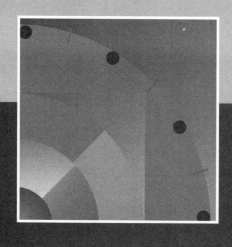

Contributors

The following nurses and health care providers contributed tips and timesavers for this chapter:

Kathryn E. Ausprung, RN, BSN

Jennie Brown, LPN

Dianne Charron, RN

Wendy Dabney, RN

Cathy Farmer, RNC

Linda S. Fish, RN, BSN

Rita A. Fleming, RN

Marcy Portnoff Gever, RPH, MED

Myra Horn, RN

Jacqueline Jeffries, RN, BSN

Wendy Kaveney, RN, BSN

Carolyn Kross, RN

Melissa Lebon, RN

Emoke Lukacs, RN

Diane Lyness, BSN

Patricia McShane, RN

Christine M. McGrath, RN

Susan R. Potts, RN

Terrilynn M. Quillen, RN

Sandy Ringwall, RN

Cindy Sanders, RN

Sylvia Spearr, RN

Patty Swetnam, RN

J. Thuman, RN

Patricia Trefethen, RN

Rose Marie Utley, RN, CPNP

Diane Voellner, RN, MN

Cathy L. Wilt, LPN

Fluid and nutrition

DOWN THE SPOUT
Getting bedridden children to drink may cause more fluid to be spilled than consumed, especially with tots who haven't quite mastered drinking through straws or who aren't allowed straws. Eliminate the mess by using special drinking cups—the kind that have a sipper lid. They can be found in most grocery stores or drugstores. So, if a child can raise his head, he can drink—unassisted and unafraid of spilling.

CIRCUITOUS SOLUTION
Getting small children to force fluids can be a problem. Use plastic "crazy straws," which are constructed in complicated shapes. The youngsters love watching the path of the juice when they sip. They take adequate fluids and won't let the straw out of sight.

Play therapy

PUT UP A HAPPY FACE
To increase visual stimulation for infants who require restraint (such as those undergoing cleft lip repair), tape pictures of happy, smiling faces inside their cribs (toothpaste advertisements in magazines work especially well). The little ones seem to enjoy gazing at human faces.

BOUNCY MOBILE
Here's a way to make a colorful, inexpensive mobile to stimulate infants and bedridden youngsters. Punch eight holes in a paper or Styrofoam dinner plate, making a circular pattern. Cut a long piece of string into four 24" (60 cm) pieces; then thread each piece up through the bottom of the plate and down through the next hole.

Now you can be creative. Cut animal pictures from magazines, or make snowflakes or other shapes from colored paper, and tie your creations to the strings hanging from the plate. To suspend the mobile, just punch two more holes in the center of the plate, and thread a strong rubber band through the holes, tying it to a long string at the top. Then tape the string to the ceiling or hang it from an I.V. pole.

The rubber band makes the animals and snowflakes dance if the child pulls on the mobile, and it gives the plate some bounce so it won't tear easily.

WATER PLAY FOR HAND BURNS

Here's a first-aid suggestion for relieving minor hand burns in young patients.

Advise parents to keep some colored, plastic ice cube containers, preferably the kind shaped like letters or numbers, in the freezer. If a child burns his hand, place the cubes in a bowl of cool water and tell the child to "catch" the shapes.

INVENTIVE INCENTIVES

Need some incentive to get your pediatric patients to use incentive spirometers or practice breathing exercises? Try the following techniques:
• Have the patient blow bubbles. If a toy store bubble kit isn't handy, make your own: Make a loop out of one end of a pipe cleaner. Dip the loop into some diluted baby shampoo. Then ask the child to take a deep breath and blow into the loop. He'll love the bubbles—and you'll love his sudden compliance with breathing exercises.
• Attach a surgical glove to the top of a 60-ml syringe. Have the patient put the tip of the syringe in his mouth. Then encourage him to blow up the glove. He'll enjoy counting each finger as it blows up with air. (Of course, you should closely monitor the child when he practices this or any other breathing exercise.)
• Wrap some thin paper (such as onionskin typing paper or tissue paper) around a comb. Give the comb to the child and ask him to "make music" by blowing on it.

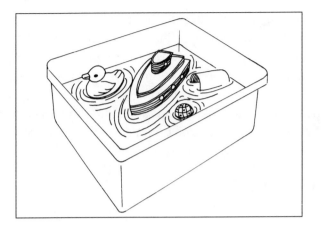

MAKING FINGER SOAKS FUN
My 2-year-old son resisted warm finger soaks for cellulitis—until I added plastic toys to the water. Then he played happily while complying with the doctor's order.

PINWHEEL POWER
Here's a way to get a child to breathe deeply so you can auscultate his lungs. Give him a colorful pinwheel to play with. You can auscultate his lungs as he takes deep breaths to make the wheel spin.

A DOLL OF A PATIENT
Trying to get a 2-year-old to take medicine can be a real battle. Before a child has to take antibiotics or cough medicine, pretend to give some to a doll. After watching a "sick" dolly take the medicine, the child may take his dose more willingly.

Procedures

INFANT BLOOD SPECIMENS
To get a sufficient amount of blood from an infant for a specimen, hold his feet in warm water for 5 to 10 minutes. (Better still, let his parents do the soak.) Then, with just one stick you should be able to obtain an adequate specimen.

INFANT CHEST PHYSIOTHERAPY

Because my hand is too big, I experienced difficulty performing chest physiotherapy on infants. Fortunately, a colleague taught me this technique: Use a pediatric resuscitation mask as a percussor. Simply cover the opening that attaches to the tubing with a piece of gauze. Alternatively, use a nipple from a baby bottle as a percussor. Before you begin, put a light blanket or diaper over the infant so the mask valve or nipple won't irritate tender skin.

BRIGHT SOCKS FOR BABY

When suctioning an infant at home, put brightly colored socks on his hands. This will distract him, so you won't have active hands in your way.

A COLLECTOR'S ITEM

Need to get a urine specimen from an infant or toddler? Apply a pediatric urine collection bag. But if you put a diaper over the bag, you risk squeezing the bag and causing the baby discomfort as well as having urine leak out. A safer, more comfortable alternative is this:

Make a large X-shaped slash in the diaper at the front of the crotch. Place the collection bag and diaper on the baby, and gently pull the bag out through the X-shaped opening. This way, there's no pressure on the bag, and you can readily see when the baby has voided.

COLLECTING URINE WITH A CONDOM CATHETER

We designed a urine collection system for male infants and small boys that works really well. Here's what we do:

First, we place a small condom catheter over the infant's penis. Then, we cut a hole in the center of a large transparent dressing and place the dressing over the penis so that the edges of the condom are secured at the base of the penis. We reinforce the dressing with several strips of transparent dressing (cut lengthwise) by wrapping the strips around the base of the condom to create a seal. Finally, we connect a urine drainage system to the condom catheter and tape it securely.

This system lasts for 12 hours without leaking, but comes off easily after it's soaked in water. Plus, it eliminates the need to sedate the patient or use an invasive procedure.

FLAVOR LIP SAVER

If a child won't let you apply ice to his swollen lip, offer him a flavored ice pop instead. He'll probably be more receptive to the treat than to the ice.

HELPING DISABLED CHILDREN WALK

Here's something you can recommend to parents of a handicapped child: Make a set of sturdy, economical parallel bars from wooden dowels and ordinary kitchen chairs. Here's how:

Buy two 8' (2.4 m) dowels, 1" (2.5 cm) in diameter (ask for them at your local lumber yard). Sand and varnish them and attach a piece of clothesline to each end with a small nail.

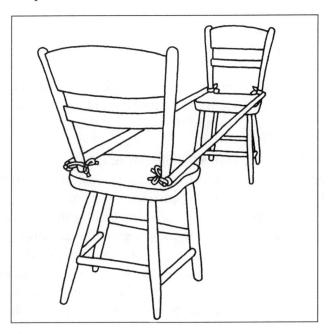

Then place the dowels on the seats of two kitchen chairs and tie the ends of the dowels to the chair backs. The height and width of the chair seats is just right for a toddler.

When the bars aren't being used, they can be untied and put away.

EAR IRRIGATION

Once, one of my young patients became terribly frightened when I tried to use a traditional irrigation syringe to clean his ear. Now, when working with children, I use a 20-ml syringe with an I.V. plastic cannula attached instead. This syringe is softer, more pliable, and less frightening to young patients than a traditional irrigation syringe.

HUGS RATHER THAN PRESSURE

I find that most preschoolers become anxious when they hear the words "blood pressure." So when I take a child's blood pressure, I simply show him the cuff (colorfully decorated) and say, "I need to give your arm a gentle hug with this arm band." I explain that I'll "listen" to his arm with my stethoscope. As I inflate the cuff, I say, "There's that hug."

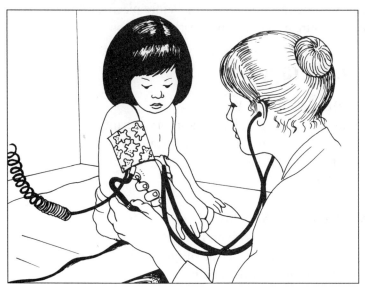

Because the child relaxes, I get a more accurate reading. Many children ask, "Can we do it again?"

SECURE SOAKS

Here's a quick and easy way to secure a warm soak against a child's arm or leg:

Put the wet dressing in place and wrap a disposable diaper with the absorbent side against the dressing snugly around it. Then secure the diaper and dressing with the diaper's adhesive tabs.

The diaper will conform to any shape, shield against wetness, retain warmth, and allow the child to move freely. You can even draw funny faces on the outside of the diaper with a felt-tip marker.

HIP-SPICA CAST CLEANLINESS

For a child with a hip-spica cast who isn't toilet trained, tuck a folded diaper under the perineal edges of the cast (around the crotch area). To hold the diaper in place, fasten a second diaper around the cast.

If the child is toilet trained, insert plastic wrap under the edges of the cast's perineal area before placing him on a bedpan. Be sure to remove the plastic after cleaning the child.

I.V. therapy

GREATER EASE WITH I.V.s

I find that starting an I.V. on a squirming infant can be tricky, so I tape his arm or leg to an armboard first. Securing the catheter after cannulation is easier if the arm is already immobilized.

KEEPING A CHILD'S I.V. INTACT

A pediatric patient with an I.V. in the antecubital fossa may have difficulty remembering not to bend his elbow. I've found that this tip works well:

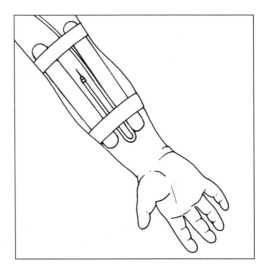

Place a tongue blade vertically on each side of the site. Then place a piece of tape horizontally across the top and bottom of both tongue blades. You'll still be able to check his I.V., but he won't be able to bend his arm.

Medications

BY THE BOTTLE

Sometimes administering medication to an infant can be very difficult—even with the aid of special spoons and syringes. Here's an easier way.

Put the medication in the baby's bottle and add water to make 1 oz (30 ml). (Check first to see if the medication can be diluted in water.) Use a regular nipple for clear medications such as cough medicines and acetaminophen drops; use a crosscut nipple with larger holes for unclear medications that are more viscous.

You can add more water to any medication left in the bottle and make sure the baby drinks it all. Don't mix medication with formula, milk, or juice because of the risk of a drug incompatibility.

GIVING INJECTIONS: HOLD STEADY
I've found a good way to give a child an I.M. injection: Have him sit on the edge of the bed, his legs slightly apart. Ask one of his parents to stand between the child's legs and hug him. The parent should keep his or her arms over the child's arms. When you give the injection, the child can't see the needle. He's securely restrained, and he has the extra comfort of holding onto Mom or Dad.

DISTRACTION TACTIC
Here's how I take the "sting" out of pediatric injections. Before I give the injection, I hand the child an adhesive bandage and ask him to cover the exact spot where the needle goes in, right after I give the shot. The child is amazed at how hard it is to find the injection site, and this distraction helps keep him calm.

"MOON GAS" MEDICATION
Here's how I help reduce a pediatric patient's fear and anxiety during an aerosol nebulizer treatment. I tell the child to pretend that he's an astronaut on a space mission and that the mask is a space mask. His goal is to withstand the "moon gas" (medication) so he can earn his flight wings. When the treatment is finished, I give him a sticker with a pair of wings on it.

EYEDROPS AND INFANTS
Giving eyedrops to a squirming infant can be especially difficult for a mother who must do it without help. Here's a tip for her:

Tell her to sit on the floor with her legs apart and to lay the baby between them with his head toward her. Then she should place his right arm under her right thigh and his left arm under her left thigh, holding his head firmly but gently between her thighs. Then she can administer the drops with both her hands while keeping his head immobilized.

FULL DOSE FOR INFANTS

Getting an infant to take an entire dose of oral medication may be difficult. I dip the outer part of a nipple in a liquid the infant likes, then I insert the medication-filled syringe into the nipple. I can administer the medication as the infant sucks, and he gets the full dose.

THE NIPPLE SOLUTION

Babies and toddlers who've had surgery are frequently given antibiotics by mouth because their I.V. lines have been discontinued. We've found a way to give these liquid medications without spills and dribbles. We cut the tip off a disposable nipple, pour the medication into the tip, and let the child suck on it. The baby gets an accurate dose, and we save time.

Patient teaching

BODY TRACINGS

Body tracings are a great tool for helping young diabetic patients learn insulin injection site rotation. Here's how to make a tracing:

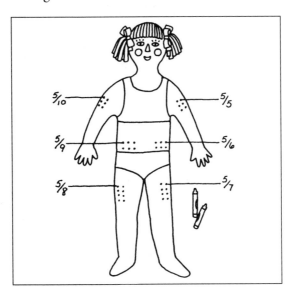

Trace the child's body outline on a large piece of brown wrapping paper. The two sides of the paper represent the front and back of the child's body. After each injection, help the child find and date the site on the paper.

The child also can decorate the tracing with yarn and felt-tip pens.

IN CASE OF POISONING, CALL FIRST

I tell a child's parents to attach the phone numbers of their local poison control center and their pediatrician to a bottle of syrup of ipecac. These phone numbers are a reminder to contact the poison control center *before* administering any treatment. Advise the parents to administer any emergency treatment recommended by the poison control center and then to contact the child's pediatrician.

MODEL FOR TRACH CARE

To teach a young patient and his family members about tracheostomy care, hollow out a foam toy football. Place the inner cannula into this hollowed-out section; then tie the trach ties around the football. Doing this will give the patient and family a feel for how the cannula should go in and come out. Leave the model with the patient and caregiver so they can practice and teach other family members.

TEACHING VENTILATION

If a baby you are caring for has a tracheostomy and occasionally needs artificial ventilation when he becomes apneic and stimulation won't arouse him, you'll need to teach his mother how to ventilate him.

To help her practice, make a model respiratory system from the following materials: two finger cots, two rubber bands, a small Y-connector, some oxygen tubing, and a trach tube. Use the Y-connector to attach the finger cots to the oxygen tubing, securing them with the rubber bands. Then attach the trach tube to the other end of the tubing. Finally, attach a hand-held resuscitation bag to the trach tube.

Now the mother can practice gauging the amount and rate of pressure needed to inflate the finger-cot "lungs."

THINK THUNDER

Several of my pediatric patients have chronic otitis media. To teach parents the signs and symptoms to watch for, I developed the acronym *THUNDER*. It stands for:
- *T*emperature
- *H*earing loss
- *U*pper respiratory infections
- *N*ausea
- *D*izziness
- *E*arache
- *R*ed ears

I remind parents that otitis media feels like "thunder" in their child's ears, and I write the signs and symptoms on an index card for them to keep as a reference.

WARNING SIGNS

I advise parents to consult their child's doctor if any of the following persist or recur:
- fever
- pain
- pallor
- lump or thickening anywhere on the body
- changes in gait
- personality changes
- eye changes (physical or visual).

The presence of one or more of these signs in a child *may* indicate cancer. Note that cancer warning signs in children are distinct from adult warning signs.

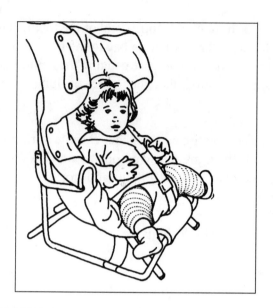

CAR SEAT SAFETY

A child wearing a Pavlik harness or hip-spica cast may not fit into a standard car seat. In such cases, I advise parents to ask their doctor or hospital social service office about making modifications to the car seat. For example, the plastic bucket of the seat might be cut to accommodate a hip-spica cast, as shown.

To ensure safety, a reputable testing organization should evaluate the crashworthiness of a modified seat.

Legal issues

CHILD ABUSE

Two years ago, I suspected a child under my care was being abused. On two home visits, I found multiple bruises on his arm and leg, and his mother could offer only vague explanations as to what happened. I contacted the department of social welfare (the agency in my state empowered to investigate acts of abuse). During this experience, I learned some important facts about reporting child abuse:

• A federal law, the Child Abuse Prevention and Treatment Act of 1973, protects you from liability; if you file the report in good faith, this law will protect you from any suit filed by an alleged abuser. Most state child abuse laws will also protect you from liability related to reporting actual or suspected abuse.

• In many states, failure to report actual or suspected abuse constitutes a crime. Not filing a report can have more serious consequences than filing one that contains an unintentional error.

• Abuse raises many difficult emotional issues. However, I had to make my report to authorities as complete, objective, and accurate as possible. Once I decided to file the report, I could not let my feelings affect the content of my report.

6

The Maternal and Neonatal Patient

Contents

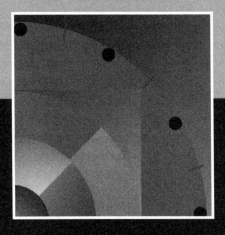

Contributors

The following nurses provided tips and timesavers for this chapter:

Kay J. Bandell, RN

Dawn Denton, RN

Donald M. Grubb, RN, MSN, ARNP

Bonnie Handerhan, RN, BSN

Teresa Hays, RN

Denise Houle, RN

Susan Lea, RN

Janet E. Marshman, RN

Marie M. Savoie, BSN

Maureen A. Storey, RN

Barbara J. Whitmore, RN

Muriel A. Zraning, RN

Prenatal care

PREECLAMPSIA POINTS

Pregnancy-induced hypertension is a potentially life-threatening illness. When assessing prenatal patients during home visits, I always check for the following signs:
• swelling of face, hands, legs, and feet
weight gain of 2 lb (0.9 kg) or more a day
• headaches
• dizziness
• blurred vision
• shimmering vision
• spots before the eyes
• right upper quadrant pain
• decreased fetal movement.

   If my patient experiences any of these, I notify her doctor immediately.

BREAST APPEARANCE

Assessing pregnant women as part of home care? Expect to see large or pendulous breasts. Other normal breast findings will include enlarged, erectile nipples; colostrum secretion; dark, broadened areolae; prominent Montgomery tubercles; vascular bluish chest veins; and striae from stretching.

BREAST PALPATION

While palpating the breasts of a pregnant patient, don't be alarmed if you note a discharge; this is a normal finding.

Breast-feeding

NUMB MUM

A new mother who wants to breast-feed her baby but whose nipples are sore might appreciate this suggestion.

   Just before breast-feeding, tell her to wrap some ice chips in a cloth and apply it to the nipple. In a minute or so, the nipple will be numb, the baby can start sucking, and the mother won't feel the soreness that usually accompanies the first few moments of breast-feeding. (Cold also makes the nipple more erect, so it's easier for baby to grasp.)

HELPING A BABY BREAST-FEED

I once provided home care to a new mother who experienced difficulty breast-feeding her baby because her nipples weren't large enough to induce the sucking response.

To help out, I cut a regular disposable nipple in half lengthwise and placed part of it on top of the mother's nipple. The nipple provided enough stimulation to help the baby suck. The mother held onto the nipple until her baby began nursing; then she gently pulled it away.

This technique allowed her to breast-feed her baby and ended her frustration.

NURSING REMINDER

A nursing mother should alternate breasts each time she begins to breast-feed her baby. To help her remember which breast to use for the start of her baby's next feeding, suggest she put a small safety pin on the cup of her bra. After each feeding, she should move the pin to the other side to remind her to start with the other breast next time.

THE PERFECT MODEL

My colleagues and I needed a breast model to teach new mothers about breast-feeding. The model had to be portable, pliable, realistic, *and* inexpensive. A small, inflated, oblong balloon met all these criteria.

The end of the balloon represents a nipple. (Or if we want to show a flat nipple, we hold the inflated balloon in the middle and force the air to the end.) We can demonstrate nipple preparation exercises and how to use a breast pump on our balloon breast model. And we always get a laugh when we pull out a green, orange, or multicolored breast model.

EASING MASTITIS

Mastitis makes breast-feeding uncomfortable, but it doesn't mean a mother must stop breast-feeding her baby. In fact, breast-feeding can speed her recovery. Here are three tips to increase comfort:

• Feed baby as often as he is hungry; frequent breast emptying prevents milk from accumulating and allowing bacterial growth.

• Wear a comfortable bra for support, but make sure it's not too tight.

• Apply heat or cold to the breast to reduce pain; try a warm moist washcloth, warm shower, cold moist washcloth, or ice pack.

SORE NO MORE

Breast-feeding doesn't have to lead to sore, cracked nipples— not if the new mom takes a few minutes each day to prevent them.

Here's what I recommend: Use water only to clean the breasts and gently rub the nipples with a terry cloth towel once or twice a day for about 30 seconds, ideally right after bathing.

Postpartum care

COOL COMFORT

For my postpartum patient, I put perineal pads in the refrigerator. When they're cool, I take one out, sprinkle it with cold water, place it next to the perineum, and then apply an ice pack. The cool pad comforts her sore perineum and protects her skin from the ice pack.

CONTROLLED RELAXATION

The controlled-relaxation techniques for labor and delivery taught in prepared childbirth classes can be used prenatally and postpartum, too. For example, women who have difficulty falling asleep during late pregnancy may find that controlled relaxation helps induce sleep in a short time.

Also, nursing mothers who are tense or nervous at feeding times may find that controlled relaxation works better than a glass of wine or beer.

POSTPARTUM POINTERS
To assess a postpartum patient who's had a vaginal delivery, remember the phrase: *For Every Lady Be Vigilant.* It'll remind you to check the following assessment parameters:
• *Fundus*
• *Episiotomy site*
• *Lochia*
• *Breasts*
• *Voiding.*

POSTPARTUM PADS
If your postpartum patient is breast-feeding her baby, she may appreciate this tip:

Instead of commercial bra pads, try using beltless sanitary minipads. Simply cut a minipad in half, peel the backing off both halves, and affix one half to each side of the bra.

The minipad halves are highly absorbent and have a stay-dry lining that helps prevent irritated nipples and leaking. Besides, they're much cheaper—less than half the cost of most commercial bra pads.

COOL PAD
Here's a method of applying ice to a patient's perineum after an episiotomy:

First, cut a sanitary pad in half—the short way—and soak the halves in water until saturated. Then take each half and fashion it into a 1" (2.5-cm) diameter roll. Next, cover each roll with a 5" × 5" (12.7 cm × 12.7 cm) square of plastic kitchen wrap and put it into the freezer.

When the roll is frozen, place one or two witch hazel (Tucks) pads on the patient's perineum, put one or both of the frozen rolls over the Tucks pads, and hold both roll and pads in place with another whole sanitary pad.

Neonatal care

PROTECTING A BABY'S SKIN

A young infant who's had surgery may need frequent dressing changes. Because the tape used to secure the dressing could excoriate the baby's fragile skin, here is an alternative.

Lay the baby on an open surgical mask; then loosely cross and tie the straps of the mask over the dressing. To change the dressing, gently untie the straps. You now have easy access to the wound without harming the skin.

PRINTED POINTERS FOR PARENTS

A new mother receives a lot of information (such as breast-feeding and car safety films, bath demonstrations, nutrition lectures) in a short period of time—especially if she's discharged within 48 hours after delivery. It's no wonder, then, that she's overwhelmed with all these new facts, figures, and explanations.

My colleagues and I made up a folder to give to the mother on the first home visit that contains information, on parenting. It includes information on resources such as the La Leche League and a sheet with practical information, such as cord care, how to take the baby's temperature, and what to do if the baby is fussy, has diarrhea, or is vomiting. We also include a sheet describing the mother's physical condition during the postpartum period. New mothers appreciate the folder because it reinforces what was already discussed with them during their short stay in the hospital.

BIKINI DIAPER

For a neonate who needs phototherapy, try making a bikini diaper using a four-stringed, disposable face mask with the metal nosepiece removed. This mini-diaper allows maximum skin exposure to the lights while protecting the neonate's genitals.

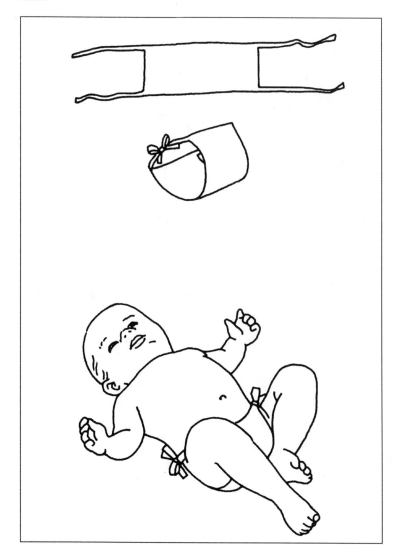

A FULL FEEDING

Newborns tend to tire easily, especially newborns with heart and lung problems. Tired infants have trouble nursing from a bottle long enough to get a full feeding. My recommendation to parents: Use a nipple designed for premature babies or one with large holes. This will allow the infant to feed more easily.

SLIPPERY BUSINESS

Sinks, tubs, and plastic baby tubs are all too slippery for bathing a wiggling, protesting newborn. The safest and easiest way, the one I suggest to new moms and dads: Give baby a sponge bath at first.

Then, when he's 6 weeks old or so, line a sink or baby tub with a large towel or piece of foam to prevent baby from slipping, and introduce him to his first bath. Refrain from using a full-sized tub until baby can sit up.

Remind the parents: *Never, never* leave a baby of any age alone in or near the sink, tub, or baby bath.

PREVENTING DIAPER RASH

Have the parents of an infant with diaper rash been told to expose his red, sore buttocks to room air? To do so and still

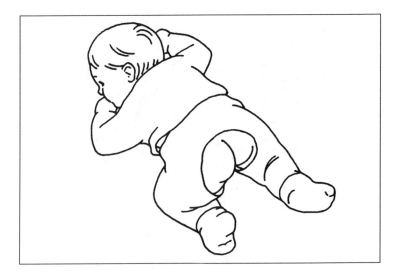

keep the infant warm, I recommend that they put a second undershirt on the baby, according to the following directions.

Put the first undershirt on as usual; then, put the second on so the infant's legs go through the arms of the undershirt. Leave the buttocks exposed through the neck opening.

APNEA MONITORING

When a newborn needs apnea monitoring, here's what I teach parents:

• Place the electrode belt over the infant in line with the nipples.

• Electrodes should touch the infant's skin.

• Make sure that the leadwires lead away from the infant's skin, face, and neck.

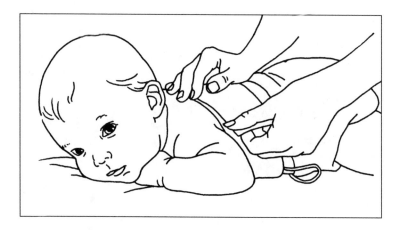

7

Patient Teaching

Contents

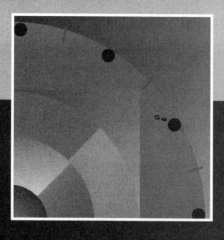

Contributors

The following nurses and health care providers provided tips and timesavers for this chapter:

Maureen Anthony, RN

Elisa B. Bachrow, LPN

Arline M. Brice, SN

Sandra Dearholt, RN, CCRN, BSN

Diane Deegan-McCrann, RN, ET

Marion B. Dolan, RN

Mary Jo Early, RN

Donna Eichna, RN, CS, MSN

Angie Fuller, RN, BSN

Teresa Gentry, RN, BSN

Theresa Gilliland, RN

John Hamby, PhD

Corinne C. Harmon, RN, MS

Joyce E. Heil, RN, BSN

Stacy C. Hoffman, SN

Carol I. Lewis, RN

Diana McLeod, RN

Tammy Mertes, SN

Gale Nunn, RN

Kirsten Rutherford-Harris, RN

Teresa Ryan, RN

Eileen M. Suraci, RN

Elissa Sommer, RN

Marjorie B. Shaljean, RN

Amy Swango, RN, MSN

Julie R. Welsh, RN, MS

Joan Woods, RN

Promoting health

STROKE WARNING SIGNS

When teaching my patients the warning signs of a possible stroke, I find this mnemonic helpful: *We k*N*ow the* H*ints of a Possible Stroke. We can* S*ee the* D*ifference.*

The phrase helps my patients remember to be on the lookout for:
- *Weakness*
- *Numbness*
- *Headache*
- *Personality changes*
- *Speech changes*
- *Sight changes*
- *Dizziness.*

INFECTION DETECTION

To help patients remember the signs of infection to report to the doctor, just remind them that "*People* S*hould* R*eally* H*elp People.*" Then teach them the following signs:
- *Pain*
- *Swelling*
- *Redness*
- *Heat*
- *Pus.*

TEACHING WITH TRIM

My colleagues and I have adopted a teaching method known by the acronym "TRIM" to help make sure our patients can care for themselves between visits. This method helps standardize patient teaching and encourages patients to understand and remember the components of their care.

How does it work? As an example, here's what we tell a patient with congestive heart failure:
- *Treatment:* Check weight weekly.
- *Restrictions:* Eliminate salt and salted foods. Avoid extremes

of heat, humidity, and cold. Don't exercise strenuously; however, you should walk 1 mile a day. Schedule daily rest periods.
• *I*mpending signs and symptoms: Report swelling of hands or feet, shortness of breath, or weight gain of 3 pounds (1.36 kg) or more per week to your doctor.
• *M*edications: Digoxin, 0.25 mg, four times a day; furosemide, 40 mg, twice a day; potassium chloride, 30 mEq, four times a day. Take all medications as directed. Report any adverse reactions to your doctor.

RISK REDUCTION REMINDERS

I've devised this mnemonic to teach patients how to reduce risk of atherosclerosis:
• *R*ed meat should be limited to 3 to 4 ounces (115 to 113 g) a day.
• *E*xercise or engage in daily activity.
• *D*o listen to your doctor.
• *U*se less salt while cooking or at the table.
• *C*holesterol should be maintained within appropriate range for age and sex (normal range is 170 to 200 mg/dl).
• *E*at less fried food and more vegetables.

STRATEGY FOR TEACHING RELAXATION

Many patients are skeptical about the efficacy of relaxation techniques, such as guided imagery, meditation, and deep breathing, in helping to control pain.

I find it best to begin teaching relaxation techniques while the patient has minimal or no pain. I encourage regular practice and try to provide plenty of time for patients to become skilled at relaxation techniques before pain worsens. This strategy helps boost the patient's confidence that relaxation techniques will work.

I try to find out what practice method is suitable for each patient. Some patients feel less self-conscious if you practice alongside them. Others prefer to practice in private. Encourage your patient to practice in whatever manner is comfortable for him. If need be, help the patient find a quiet room to practice relaxation techniques without distractions.

ALLERGY-PROOFING STRATEGIES
Here are tips I offer my home care patients to help them reduce exposure to allergens and thereby reduce symptoms:
• Clear your bedroom of dust catchers, such as knickknacks, stuffed animals, wall hangings, and books.
• Use blankets made of synthetic materials rather than wool.
• Replace feather pillows and comforters with those filled with Dacron, nylon, or other polyester fibers.
• Encase your mattress or boxspring in airtight vinyl covers.
• Remove plants and aquariums from your bedroom because these may increase mold spores in the air.
• Dust at least two or three times weekly. Use a damp mop or cloth instead of a broom, which can raise dust.
• Use an electronic air cleaner to remove mold, house dust, and pollens from the air. Be sure to wash or replace the filter periodically.
• In warm weather, close the windows and use an air conditioner.
• Clean air-conditioner and heater outlets regularly.

Customizing your teaching

NOT BY THE WRITTEN WORD
During my home care visits, I occasionally encounter patients who experience difficulty reading. Here are strategies I use to foster learning:
• Draw pictures that illustrate teaching lessons, making sure the most important points are clearly highlighted.
• Tape-record instructions and encourage the patient to play them back until he's memorized necessary information.
• Ask the patient to repeat instructions after giving them orally.
   I've also noticed that some of my colleagues have a tendency to shout when speaking to illiterate patients. I try to

remind them to speak in a normal voice. Just because a patient can't read doesn't mean he can't hear you.

UNDERSTANDING A "NO SEEDS" DIET
A simple analogy explains why a patient with diverticulosis can't eat seeds. I compare a seed getting caught in the intestines with a seed getting caught under the dentures. The patient can understand the pain, inflammation, and possible infection that might cause. And I tell him that although he could remove the dentures and seed, treatment for a seed lodged in the intestines isn't as easy.

This analogy isn't 100% medically accurate, but it's quickly grasped and helps reinforce the "no seeds" diet.

CUSTOMIZED MEDICATION CARDS
Create customized medication cards for your patients who take several medications. It will help you and your patient keep track of prescriptions and dosages. Just type your patient's medication information in neat columns, reduce the list to business-card size by using a copy machine, and then laminate the card with self-laminating sheets.

Encourage your patient to keep the card in his wallet.

Drug	Dosage	Indication
Zestril	20 mg-1 tab-a.m.	blood pressure
Norvasc	5 mg-½ tab-p.m.	blood pressure
aspirin	81 mg-1 tab-a.m.	blood thinner
Minitran patch	0.2 mg/hr on a.m.- off p.m.	heart
Nitrostat	$\frac{1}{150}$ gr-1 tab under tongue, p.r.n.	chest pain

HEALTH HOMEWORK

Patient teaching can be a challenge if you're giving a lot of information in a limited amount of time. Here's what I do to enhance my teaching:

Before I give a patient his education pamphlet, I underline the important information in red ink. Then I tell him that his homework is to read the material so we can discuss it the next visit. If I'm demonstrating a procedure to the patient, I ask him to practice before I meet with him again.

Presenting the material as a homework assignment stresses the importance of learning. It also makes the patient more responsible for his own care.

SAY IT WITH FLOWERS

If you ever have to explain collateral circulation to a myocardial infarction patient and his family, compare your patient's injured vessel to the stem of a plant that's been accidentally broken off. When placed in a glass of water and given some time and care, the stem will sprout new roots. So, too, the patient's heart with proper care and rest will sprout new vessels.

Not only does this explanation bring a difficult subject into clearer focus, but it also gives the patient some much-needed hope for recovery.

Teaching self-care

SKIN DEBRIDEMENT AT HOME

If your home health care patient has a hand-held shower head, he can debride a leg ulcer himself. Here's how:

Tell the patient to hold the nozzle of the shower head about 6" (15 cm) from his ulcer and run warm water over it for 5 minutes. (If he has a shower chair, he might want to sit on it for comfort.)

He should do this twice a day until his ulcer heals. Of course, he should discontinue treatment if it causes pain.

PREVENTING URINE BACKFLOW

If your patient has a urinary catheter, tell him to hang the drainage bag from a mattress handle at night. This will secure the bag below his bladder, preventing urine backflow while he's sleeping. If his drainage bag can't be hooked, advise him to place it in a recyclable plastic shopping bag and tie the shopping bag around one of the mattress handles. If his mattress doesn't have handles, tell him to place the drainage bag in a large plastic bag and tuck the opening well under the mattress so that the bag dangles down.

THE RIGHT MUSCLE

To help patients manage stress incontinence, I encourage them to perform Kegel exercises to strengthen pelvic floor muscles. These exercises are performed using the following techniques:
• voluntarily stopping the stream of urine
• pulling in on rectal muscles as if retaining gas.

Here's a technique to help the patient determine if she's using the correct (pelvic floor) muscles when performing Kegel exercises. Have the patient place one hand on her abdomen while performing the exercises. If her abdomen moves, she needs to try again; she's using the wrong muscles.

AVOIDING POTASSIUM

In my practice, I care for several patients with chronic renal failure who must restrict potassium intake. It's easy to recognize and avoid most sodium-laden foods because of their salty taste, but avoiding high-potassium foods, which lack a telltale taste, is trickier. Examples of high-potassium foods include the following:
• Fruits: all dried fruits, apricot juice, bananas, cantaloupe, grapefruit, honeydew melon, and oranges
• Vegetables: all raw vegetables, leafy green vegetables, beans, legumes, potatoes, tomatoes, and winter squash
• Other: molasses, nuts, and whole grains.

Low-potassium foods include the following:
• Fruits: apples, cranberries, grapes, and pears (fresh, canned, or juice)
• Vegetables: canned carrots, corn, green beans, or peas; and fresh summer squash
• Other: honey, noodles, rice, and white enriched bread.

Teach your patient which foods he should eat and which he should avoid. Suggest that he post a list of high- and low-potassium foods on his refrigerator and check the list before eating.

DRUG RISK AWARENESS

Patients with impaired renal function face increased risk of nephrotoxic effects from drugs. For these patients, I always place special emphasis on teaching safe drug therapy. In particular, I tell them to:
• Make a list of all current medications, both prescription and nonprescription drugs.
• Inform their doctor, nurse, and other health care providers about all conditions for which they take medications.

I also make my patients aware that, although many drugs can disrupt kidney function, most problems are caused by three major groups:
• antibiotics
• nonsteroidal anti-inflammatory drugs
• contrast dyes used in diagnostic X-ray tests.

PULLEY ARM LIFT

When one of my patients has an aching shoulder, I provide instructions for an arm pulley exercise. Here's what I tell the patient to do:

Drape a bath towel over a secure shower rod or attach a pulley and rope in an open doorway. Grab one end of the towel or rope with each hand. Then, using the unaffected arm, gently pull on the towel or rope, and lift the sore arm. When you've raised your sore arm as high as you can without discomfort, hold the position for a few seconds. Then let the arm drop slowly.

SANDPAPER MED LABELS

If a blind patient is taking several medications in tablet form and wants to take them by himself, try this system developed by one of my patients:

Begin by cutting letters and numbers out of sandpaper. Using the sandpaper letters, label seven envelopes with the days of the week. Then, using the sandpaper numbers, label small self-sealing plastic bags according to the time the tablets are to be taken. Place the tablets in the plastic bags, put the bags inside the envelopes, and file them in a shoe box within the patient's reach.

Each morning, the patient simply pulls the first envelope from the box, "reads" the numbers on the plastic bags with his fingers, and takes his tablets at the designated hours.

This system not only fosters the patient's independence, but also gives you an accurate way to tell whether he's taken all of his medications.

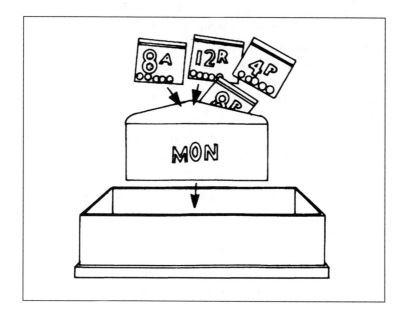

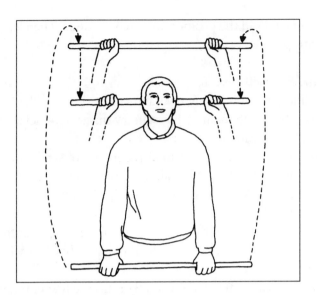

BROOMSTICK EXERCISE
Many of my patients report success with an exercise I teach them to ease aching shoulders. Here's how it works:

Grasp a broomstick (or cane or yardstick) with both hands and hold it at hip level. Then lift the stick over your head, and lower it behind your head to the back of your neck. Hold this position for as long as comfortable. Each day, try to hold the broomstick behind your head a little longer until you can hold it for several minutes.

PROTECTIVE GARMENTS
If your patient is beginning a bladder retraining program, she may experience intermittent dribbling. So I suggest that my patients wear a protective garment or pad, such as a thin panty liner or light sanitary pad. This will keep her dry, comfortable, and feeling more secure.

BLADDER ALARM
If you are working with a patient on a bladder retraining program, consider this tip: Tell the patient to set an alarm clock or kitchen timer to remind him when to use the toilet.

KNEE CARE MEMORY AID

When one of my patients injured his knee, I used the mnemonic, RICE, to help him remember the stages in knee care: *R*est, *I*ce, *C*ompression, and *E*levation. Here's how it works:
• *R*est the knee by staying off it at least 24 hours.
• Apply *I*ce for 20 minutes every half hour for a day or longer.
• Use a *C*ompression device such as an elastic bandage or brace to support the injured tissues and reduce swelling.
• *E*levate the knee above heart level to control swelling.

SELECTING A SUPPLEMENT

If your patient is advised to take an over-the-counter calcium supplement, he may become overwhelmed by the variety of supplements available. Here are some guidelines to help the patient choose a suitable supplement:
• Check product labels for the amount of elemental calcium (the amount of calcium the body actually uses); the patient should find out from his doctor how much supplemental calcium he needs.
• Avoid dolomite and bone meal preparations, which may contain lead.
• Be aware that calcium carbonate supplements may cause gas and constipation. Drinking more fluids and increasing fiber intake between meals may reduce these effects.

EXPEDIENT EXTRACT

Many of my patients have complained that the liquids and tablets for deodorizing ostomy appliances are costly and don't always work that well. I recommend vanilla extract as an inexpensive, effective alternative. Instruct patients to saturate a small wad of tissue with vanilla extract and place it in the bottom of the appliance. They can repeat this procedure as often as necessary—every time they empty the appliance, if they desire.

COLOSTOMY CLEANING TIP #1
Cleaning a colostomy or ileostomy pouch can be difficult for a home health care patient. I tell my patients to purchase a small plastic squirt bottle (they are inexpensive and available at any drugstore) that has a screw-on top. The patient can carry the bottle in his jacket pocket and fill it with tap water when needed. This way he'll be able to keep the pouch clean, no matter where he is.

COLOSTOMY CLEANING TIP #2
To reduce the odor from a colostomy bag, tell the patient to add some mouthwash to the water he uses to rinse the bag. Also tell the patient to put a small amount of mouthwash in the bag before he closes it.

COLOSTOMY CLEANING TIP #3
Here's a tip for your patient with a colostomy: Suggest he spray the inside of his colostomy bag with a cooking oil spray (such as Pam) before applying the bag. His stools won't stick to the bag, and cleanup will be easier.

FILTERING STONES
Here's a tip for your patients who must strain their urine for renal calculi or gravel. Advise them to use a cone-shaped filter for an automatic coffee maker as a handy urine strainer. The filters are small-pored and can be easily handled and disposed of. Also, if the patient passes any blood that's not readily visible, a pink or red stain will appear on the white filter paper.

DRESSING CHANGES
Here's an instruction hint for patients who need just a small dressing or protective cover for their incision after they're discharged: Apply a sanitary pad with an adhesive strip to the undergarment covering the incision. The pad protects the incision and is more economical than a sterile dressing.

Because the adhesive strip is attached to the garment, there is no adhesive touching the skin to irritate the sensitive surgical site.

Teaching the diabetic patient

MAGNIFIED MENUS

At our home care agency, we instruct diabetic patients on meal planning. When we copy printed literature on the subject to give to our patients, we adjust the copier to increase the print size. Since many diabetics have poor eyesight, this helps them read the information that's so important to our teaching.

DIABETES STREET TALK

For some patients, my colleagues and I use analogies to explain the pathophysiology of diabetes. We tell them to think of the body's blood vessels as streets, the cells as garages, the sugar as cars, and insulin as the driveways that allow cars to get from the streets into the garages.

In Type I, insulin-dependent diabetes, the pancreas doesn't produce the insulin needed to carry sugar from the blood into the cells. The analogy for the patient: The cars (sugar) stay on the street (blood vessels) because there aren't any driveways (insulin).

In Type II, non-insulin-dependent diabetes, where insulin is produced but meets resistance at the cellular level, we use this analogy: The driveways (insulin) are there, but the garage doors (cells) are closed. Because there's too much fat inside the cells, only so many cars (sugar) will fit into the garages (cells). The rest stay on the streets (blood vessels).

IMPROVISING AN INJECTION GUIDE

Recently, I was teaching a blind diabetic patient how to administer her insulin. When practicing, she'd often miss the

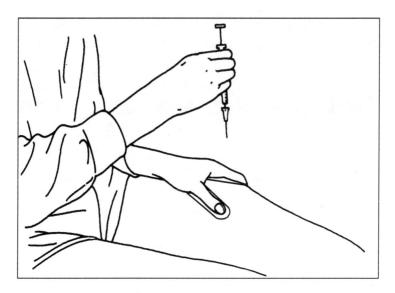

injection site and stick her fingers (which were holding the skin taut) instead.

So I made an injection guide by taping two tongue blades together at one end to form a V. Then, just before she was ready to inject herself, she placed the tongue blades on her thigh, felt the outline of the blades, and inserted the needle— right on target—inside the V.

PRACTICE PAD #1

Teaching a newly diagnosed diabetic patient to fill a syringe is usually easy. But teaching him to inject the insulin is another story—jabbing the needle into the skin is scary. So, to help patients learn this technique, use an injection practice pad.

Place a foam rubber sponge, measuring 6" × 8" x 1" (15 cm × 20 cm × 2.5 cm), between two sheets of clear plastic about 1" (2.5 cm) larger than the sponge. Seal the edges of the plastic with tape. Then punch holes in the reinforced edges on each end and insert strings for ties. Finally, cut a large target hole in the plastic on one side. Then tie the pad snugly around the patient's upper thigh.

Using 0.5 ml of sterile water instead of insulin, the patient can practice injecting the needle through the sponge until he learns the proper direction and force. Placing the pad on his thigh also lets him practice at an actual injection site.

PRACTICE PAD #2
To help diabetic patients become more confident about giving themselves insulin injections, try this: Fold an elastic bandage to a thickness greater than the length of an insulin syringe needle. Tape it to the patient's skin at the site where he'll give the real injection later. Let him practice "sticking" the bandage, using a sterile insulin syringe and a vial of sterile water.

PRACTICE PAD #3
Injecting needles into an orange doesn't give patients the feel of tissue penetration that accompanies real injections. Try letting them practice on uncooked chicken breasts with the skin still attached. Using a realistic model like that can better prepare them for the real thing.

ROTATION REMINDER
When teaching a newly diagnosed diabetic patient the importance of rotating injection sites, reinforce your lesson by marking the sites with a povidone-iodine swab. Since the povidone-iodine eventually washes off, give your patient a site rotation card as a *constant* reminder of his last injection site.

SERVING SIZE
When teaching diabetic patients about diet, I emphasize the importance of measuring food portions. I suggest that they make model portions out of Play-Doh to represent serving sizes of ¼, ⅓, ½, ⅔, ¾, and 1 cup. They can put these on a cookie sheet. Then, when they prepare meals, they can compare

each serving to the appropriate model to estimate the right quantity. This saves time and should be fairly accurate.

Another tip I give my patients: To cut down on consumption of salad dressing, use a separate dish for the dressing and dip each bite of salad into it, instead of pouring the dressing on the salad.

INSULIN ORDER
Here's a tip for teaching a patient to draw up fast-acting and long-lasting insulin into the same syringe. To help the patient get the order right, tell the patient to remember this phrase: *Fast first, long last.*

8

Medications

Contents

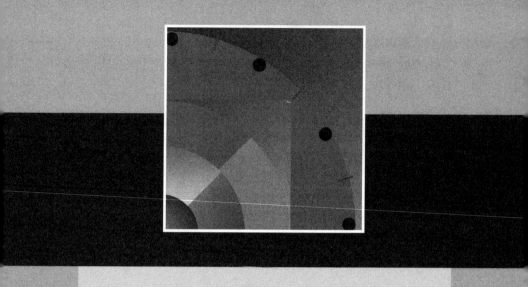

Contributors

The following nurses provided tips and timesavers for this chapter:

Leslie M. Attig, RN

Robert N. Anderson, RN, CCRN, CEN

Cathleen M. Burrage, RN, BSN

Karen Gray Pigott, RN

Oral medications

A MORE PALATABLE PILL
I've had several patients complain that aluminum hydroxide antacids taste chalky. I recommend these patients refrigerate the medication. Aluminum hydroxide antacids taste less chalky when cool, and your patient may find them more palatable.

TOUGH TO SWALLOW
When your patient has difficulty swallowing tablets, follow these guidelines:
• Don't crush the tablet and don't encourage the patient to chew it without being sure that drug delivery won't be altered. Many times, tablet coatings control when and where the medication is released into your patient's system; altering the drug may also alter its delivery mechanism and lead to improper dosing. Check with your agency or pharmacy before crushing a medication or altering it in any way.
• Try dipping the tablet or capsule in maple syrup; the sweet liquid should help the medication slide down the patient's throat.

KEEPING TRACK
Here's an easy way to avoid confusion about your patients' drug therapy: List all your patients alphabetically in a prescription notebook; then record the drugs they're taking. Encourage each patient to keep a written record as well. Such a list, when taken to the doctor or pharmacy, can help identify possible drug interactions.

MEDICATION REMINDER #1
Many of my patients take several different pills at different times a day; keeping track of the medication schedule can be bewildering. Well, I've finally discovered a way to create order out of the potential chaos (actually, I borrowed this idea from

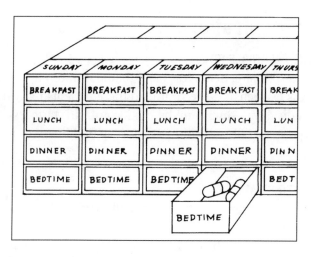

one of my patients): Make a mini-filing cabinet system. Here's what's needed and how to do it:

Get 28 cardboard sliding pill boxes, which look like matchstick boxes, from a pharmacy. Stack four boxes, one on top of another, and tape them together; stack and tape the remaining boxes in groups of four. (You should have seven stacks of four boxes each.) Place the stacks side by side and tape them together. Label the top of each stack with a day of the week. Label the four boxes in each stack "breakfast," "lunch," "dinner," and "bedtime."

Either you or your patient can fill the boxes for the upcoming week. At your next visit, you can tell by checking the boxes whether the patient's missed any medications.

MEDICATION REMINDER #2

A patient may forget a dose of a medication, especially if he has a variety of tablets and capsules to take at different times of the day. One of my home care patients, using a bulletin board, developed a clever system to remind him. Here's what he does:

First, he writes the times on separate pieces of paper and tacks them in chronological order across the top of a bulletin board. Then he writes the days of the week vertically on separate pieces of paper and tacks them on the left-hand side of the board. Next, he fills self-sealing plastic bags with the correct dose of medication for each specific time of day. (You or the patient may want to do this once a week.) Finally, he tacks the bags to the board under the appropriate day and time. He can tell at a glance when to take his medication, and he can see if he's forgotten a dose. (Special instructions, such as "Take with plenty of water," can also be attached to an appropriate spot on the bulletin board.)

The bulletin board should be kept out of reach of children and should only be used if the patient is mentally alert. Also check to make sure that the medication will not be affected by exposure to light.

EGG-XACT WAY TO REMEMBER MEDICATIONS
As a home health care nurse, I've found that many patients experience difficulty opening medicine bottles. Patients also get confused about which medication to take next. An egg carton offers a simple solution.

Label each pocket of the carton with the dosage schedule in consecutive order for 1 day. Then place the proper medication into the corresponding pocket. The cartons can be stacked so that a family member or friend can prepare medications for several days at one time.

Of course, remind the patient to keep the cartons out of the reach of children.

LET'S SPLIT
Here's a quick tip to give your patient who needs to split a tablet: Freeze the tablet for 30 minutes beforehand. Splitting it will be much easier.

NITROGLYCERIN TABLET STORAGE

A person may have trouble keeping track of his nitroglycerin tablets. Here's a way to make a convenient and safe storage place for them:

Instruct the patient to make two vertical slits in one side of an old 35 mm film container. (You can do this for him if he can't.) These slits will allow him to slide the container onto his belt. Then he can place the bottle of nitroglycerin tablets in the container and replace the lid.

Parenteral medications

TO ASPIRATE OR NOT TO ASPIRATE

Quick tip: Don't aspirate for a blood return when giving heparin or insulin. Why? Aspiration isn't necessary with insulin administration and may cause a hematoma during heparin administration.

RELAXATION IS KEY

When giving an I.M. injection, I always encourage the patient to deep breathe and relax. Most important, the patient should relax the muscle about to receive the injection. Injections into tense muscles are the most painful and cause the most bleeding.

TOE WIGGLE TECHNIQUE

One of my patients just couldn't relax for his injections. Once, I asked him to wiggle his toes. I found that wiggling helped the patient relax his muscles and momentarily distracted him from the injection.

REPEATED INJECTIONS: ICE IS NICE

Repeated injections may cause your patient pain and anxiety. Here's a technique to ease the discomfort: Numb the site with ice before cleaning it. I hold the ice in place for several seconds, then proceed as usual.

MONITORING NARCOTICS

Continuous narcotic infusions require close monitoring of a patient's breathing rate and level of alertness, especially during dosage increases.

Ensuring safe and effective home narcotic infusion therapy requires thorough training of the patient's caregiver. My advice: Encourage the caregiver to keep a diary to record information about the patient's condition. In addition to providing an important record, this will help underscore the importance of the caretaker's responsibilities.

INOTROPIC THERAPY

When providing home care to a patient with severe congestive heart failure, you may need to administer I.V. infusions of inotropic drugs, such as dopamine hydrochloride (Intropin) or dobutamine hydrochloride (Dobutrex). Pay special attention to the doctor's orders, which should state the drug's concentration, dosage in mcg/kg/min, and titration guidelines. To determine the correct dose, weigh the patient before starting therapy.

CHEMOTHERAPY

To ensure safety, certain items must be at hand before a patient can receive chemotherapy at home. Before I administer home chemotherapy, I make certain the following are available:
• clean work area for preparing the chemotherapy
• storage space for drugs and equipment
• telephone
• electricity
• refrigerator.

Diabetic medications

REUSING SYRINGES
Controversy exists surrounding the reuse of insulin syringes. Manufacturers recommend using a syringe only once. But studies suggest that some patients can use a syringe several times over a 24-hour period in certain cases.

In what situations is reuse appropriate? Research indicates that reusing insulin syringes should only be considered if the patient is meticulous in personal care and follows directions closely. Never recommend syringe reuse if the patient has poor personal hygiene, an acute illness, open wounds, or a decreased resistance to infection.

CHILLING FACTS
Here's a helpful reminder I want to share with other home care nurses: Not all insulin needs to be refrigerated. In fact, all insulins are stable at room temperature for at least a month.

Knowing this, I now tell patients to keep the vial in use at room temperature and to store unopened ones in the refrigerator to keep them stable for as long as possible.

ANGLE OF ENTRY
Experience has taught me to modify my teaching about self-injecting insulin depending on the patient's body type. For an extremely thin patient with little subcutaneous fat, I advise inserting the needle at a 45-degree angle. For an obese patient or one with a medium build, I advise inserting it at a 90-degree angle.

Miscellaneous medications

PRACTICE PASTE
Patients can practice measuring the correct dose of nitroglycerin ointment by using toothpaste instead of nitroglycerin. This is less expensive than using the actual medication. Plus,

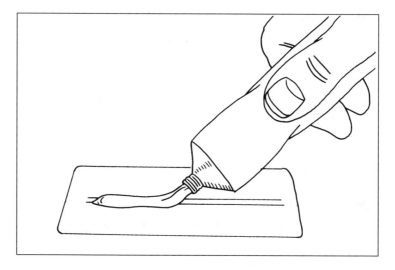

you won't have to worry about the patient possibly harming himself by getting the ointment on his fingers.

TABLETS THROUGH A TUBE

If a prescribed drug must be administered through a nasogastric tube and no liquid form is available, you will need to dissolve tablets before administration. Here's a tip: Warm water dissolves tablets more quickly and completely than cold.

SLICING SUPPOSITORIES

When I need to cut a suppository in half, I cut it lengthwise, not crosswise. Why? Suppositories are tapered, so there's less drug at the tip. Cut crosswise and the patient may receive an incorrect dose.

DON'T TOUCH

A quick reminder about using transdermal patches: I always tell my patients not to touch the gel on the patch; medication may rub off onto the patient's fingers. I also tell the patient to wash his or her hands after applying the patch; it's important to remove any medication that may have inadvertently rubbed off.

GENTLE TOUCH

Remember always to apply topical medications gently. Too much pressure can irritate a patient's skin.

HOLD YOUR BREATH

If your patient is using a medication in powder form, advise him to carefully shake the powder into his hands, then apply it to the skin. This helps protect against inhalation of airborne powder.

FOREHEAD FIRST

Here's a technique I use when applying medication to a patient's face: Start with the forehead, then spread the medication down each side of the face to the jaw, stroking in one direction only.

THE FLOATING CANISTER

Here's a way for your patient to estimate how much medication is left in an inhaler canister: Remove the canister from its plastic sleeve and place it in a large container or sink filled with water. To determine the approximate fullness of the canister, observe the extent to which it floats.

Observation	Amount in canister
Canister sinks to the bottom.	Full
Canister floats upside down near the bottom.	¾ full
Canister floats upside down and extends a quarter of the way out of the water.	½ full
Canister leans toward the surface of the water.	¼ full
Canister floats almost horizontally.	Empty

Dealing with adverse reactions

COPING WITH DRY MOUTH

When one of my patients was taking narcotic analgesics, she complained of a dry mouth. I advised her to suck on ice or sugarless candies. Encouraging her to drink adequate fluids also helped relieve the problem.

COUNTERING CONSTIPATION

Many medications, including narcotic analgesics, may cause constipation. If your patient develops constipation, recommend the following:
• high-fiber whole grain foods, such as cereals, bran products, brown rice, and whole grain breads
• fruits and vegetables
• eight to 10 eight-ounce glasses of liquid a day
• stool softener or bulk laxative, such as Metamucil.

BANISHING BRUISES

Patients on prednisone tend to bruise easily. To help prevent bruising, I tell patients to cut the feet off a pair of white sport socks and wear the socks on their arms when performing household activities. The socks, which can be hidden under long-sleeved shirts and blouses, cushion minor bumps and bangs.

PULSE CHECK

Patients on digoxin therapy are usually instructed to check their pulse before each dose. To keep track of pulse rates, I suggest they record findings in a small notebook; this provides a reminder for them and helps underscore the importance of the activity. Also I advise them to call me or their doctor if their pulse is less than 60 beats a minute.

WITHDRAW SLOWLY

If your patient is discontinuing therapy with the antihypertensive drug atenolol, monitor him carefully. The drug should be withdrawn gradually over a 2-week period to avoid serious adverse effects.

DON'T STOP SUDDENLY

Never forget to warn patients taking propranolol not to discontinue the drug suddenly. Abrupt withdrawal may exacerbate angina or cause a myocardial infarction.

9

I.V. Therapy

Contents

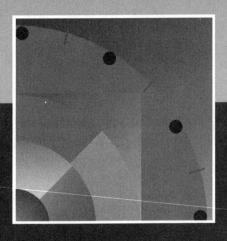

Contributors

The following nurses provided tips and timesavers for this chapter:

Beverly Anderson, RN,C, MS

Colleen Carey, RN, BSN

Ann Damore, RN, BSN

Mary Hodges, RN,C, CCRN, MS

Sonja Jones, RN

Tina L. Kipppes, RN

Sheila Ledermann, RN

Mitzi A. Llamas, RN

Terrilynn Quillen, RN

Marion Casey Renz, RN, BS

Helen Sheville, RN

Betty Woodfin, RN

Preparation and insertion

BEFORE BEGINNING

For nurses who work at my agency, performing I.V. therapy in the patient's home has become a fairly common practice. I always evaluate the following factors before starting home I.V. therapy:
• patient's age
• availability of a caregiver
• drug type, frequency of administration, and expected duration of treatment
• type of access needed
• home environment
• insurance or medicare coverage for use of I.V. equipment.

NEEDLELESS STICKS

Here's a tip to help reduce the risk of needlestick injury: Use a needleless system or a click and lock system with any type of secondary infusion or with an intermittent infusion device.

PRIMING POINT

Important reminder: Never prime an infusion system when it's connected to the patient. Do all priming before establishing any connection to the patient.

TOURNIQUET TIP

Usually, I use a flat, soft-rubber tourniquet when preparing the venipuncture site. Here's a tip I'd like to share: When applying such a tourniquet, keep it as flat as possible so that the tourniquet fits snugly but not uncomfortably.

TIME'S UP

A word of caution: Never leave a tourniquet in place for longer than 2 minutes. If you can't find a suitable vein and prepare the site within 2 minutes, remove the tourniquet. Wait a few minutes and then start again.

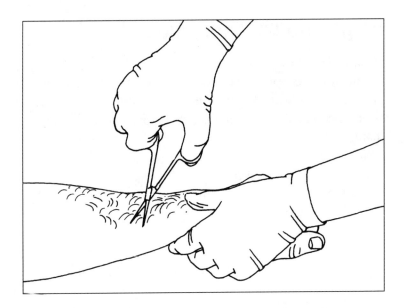

SITE PREP POINTERS

Here are a couple of pointers to help with preparing a site for venipuncture:

• To prevent skin abrasion, use scissors rather than a razor to remove hair. Avoid shaving hair at the insertion site.

• Keep in mind that the tourniquet doesn't have to be in place while you prepare the site. You may apply it after cleaning the skin.

FINDING A VEIN

Here's a tip for choosing a vein for venipuncture; aim for a round, firm, fully filled vein that rebounds when compressed. Unless the I.V. solution is very irritating, select the most distal veins first. The best veins for venipuncture are large enough to allow blood to flow around the catheter, minimizing venous irritation.

ILLUMINATING A VEIN

If you have to insert an I.V. catheter but you can't see or feel the vein, try using a penlight. Wipe both the patient's skin and the bulb end of the penlight with alcohol. Turn on the penlight and place it on the patient's skin. Look directly in front of the beam—you should see the vein. Turn off the penlight and insert the catheter as usual.

ENTERING A VEIN
Remember, you won't always feel a "pop" or sense release when a venipuncture device enters a vein. A pop usually occurs when a large-gauge needle enters a large, thick-walled vein or when the patient is a young adult.

ADVANCING ADVICE
Here's a safe way to advance an I.V. catheter: After releasing the tourniquet and removing the needle, infuse I.V. solution while advancing the catheter. This method allows rapid I.V. flow to dilate the vein and reduces the risk of puncturing the back vein wall.

BLOOD BACKFLOW
Be aware that, after inserting an I.V. device, you may not see a backflow of blood under the following circumstances:
• The device is tightly in place.
• The patient is severely dehydrated or hypovolemic.
• The device is in a small vein.

DRESSING DIRECTIONS
When using a transparent semi-permeable dressing, be careful not to stretch the dressing as you apply it. This may cause itching at the insertion site.

Ongoing care

I.V. SUPPLIES: IN THE BAG
A home health care patient requiring routine I.V. fluids can store his I.V. supplies in a clear vinyl, multi-pocket, over-the-door shoe bag. The bag takes up little space, and the vinyl is

easy to disinfect and allows the patient to see exactly where everything is. The bag is also convenient for traveling; the patient can just take it off the door, roll it up, and then unroll and hang it when he gets where he's going. Be sure to tell your patient to keep the bag away from children.

HOOKED ON HANGERS
Wire coat hangers work great as bag hooks for I.V. or enteral feeding solutions. So I advise my home health care patients with I.V. lines or enteral feeding tubes to take hangers with them on vacation. The hangers can be bent into bag hooks and then hung over doorways, closet bars, or picture frames.

TRACKING TUBING CHANGES
Changing I.V. tubing daily is a must for both intermittent and continuous therapy. To help my patients and their family members keep track of tubing changes, I suggest they label the tube with the date and time of the change.

TWIST-OFF TUBING
Here's a technique to try in case you, your patient, or the patient's caregiver has difficulty disconnecting old I.V. tubing:

Use a pair of hemostats or tweezers to hold the hub securely while you twist off the end of the tubing. To avoid damaging the tubing adapter or the venipuncture device, be careful not to clamp or squeeze too hard.

INCOMPATIBILITY INFO
When administering a drug that's incompatible with the primary I.V. solution, check with the pharmacist or drug manufacturer for directions. You may be able to take the following steps:
• Flush the line with 2 to 3 ml of 0.9% sodium chloride solution.
• Administer the drug.
• Flush the line again.

• Restart the primary I.V. solution.

If using the same I.V. line is not allowed, you'll need to insert another venipuncture device to administer the medication.

CARRY A CLAMP

Urge the patient with an external catheter, such as the Hickman catheter, to carry a catheter clamp. If the catheter is cut or begins to leak, advise him to clamp it above the leak (between the patient and the leak) to minimize blood loss. Metal clamps should be avoided because they can cut or destroy a catheter. If metal clamps are used in an emergency, a piece of gauze or even a piece of clothing between the clamp and the tubing will protect the tubing from damage.

FILTER FACTS

I.V. filters help protect the patient from hazardous microorganisms and debris that may collect in the I.V. solution. Important fact: Filters *complement* I.V. therapy; they don't replace the need for strict aseptic technique.

ATTACHING A FILTER

If you need to use a filter, always attach it to the distal end of the tubing *after* you have primed the tubing.

VOLUME CONTROL

Have you ever overfilled the chamber of a floating valve set? Here's how to remedy the situation: Immediately close the upper clamp and air vent. Then, invert the chamber and squeeze the excess fluid from the drip chamber back into the graduated fluid chamber.

INTERMITTENT INTERRUPTION

Stop immediately if you feel resistance or your patient complains of discomfort when you're flushing an intermittent infusion device. Then, check the I.V. site for swelling and redness. If either is present, remove the intermittent device and insert a new one in another site.

SHOWER CAP
Make showering easier for a patient who has a heparin lock: Cut off four of the fingers (but not the thumb) from a plastic glove. Pull the glove over the patient's hand and wrist, and secure the glove at the wrist with a piece of water-resistant tape.

THE LIGHT TOUCH
If you suspect I.V. infiltration in a patient with difficult veins, turn on a flashlight and hold it against his skin, directly over the suspicious site.

If I.V. fluid has infiltrated into the tissue, the beam will

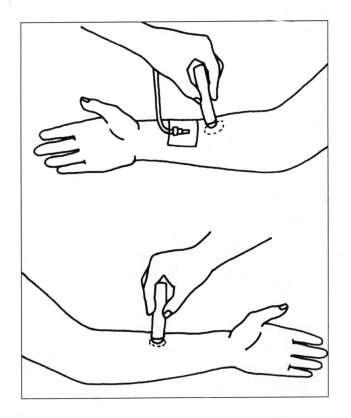

highlight the size of the infiltration. If no fluid has infiltrated, only a small halo will appear around the flashlight.

Using this trick can save you from having to do extra checks. Then, if necessary, you can stop the I.V. before the infiltration gets worse.

AVOID ALCOHOL

Quick home care tip: Don't use an alcohol sponge to clean the site when disconnecting an I.V. line. Alcohol can cause bleeding and an intense burning sensation. Instead, use a sterile gauze pad.

WEATHER WARNING

Do you provide home care for patients receiving continuous infusion therapy? If so, be prepared for the weather.

Before a severe snowstorm hits, take the following steps:
• Make sure patients who are on continuous infusions have flush kits.
• Immediately begin teaching the patient how to use the flush kit. Include in your teaching directions for disconnecting the pump and flushing the venous access device after the infusion has finished.

This way, your patients can maintain catheter patency and avoid complications until the weather clears and you can visit again.

Central venous therapy

CAP CHANGE TECHNIQUE

When changing the cap on a central venous catheter, instead of clamping the catheter, ask your patient to perform Valsalva's maneuver (unless, of course, it's contraindicated). While the patient performs Valsalva's maneuver, quickly disconnect the old cap and connect the new one.

Also, consider instructing the patient on using this technique when he changes the cap himself.

SECRETS OF CENTRAL LINE CARE

I provide care for a patient who recently returned home with a central line. Dressing changes are extremely frustrating for this patient. I advise him to use a mirror when he changes a dressing. (A small compact or makeup mirror works well.) The mirror will help him see what he's doing and allow him to check the site for signs of infection.

TRACKING FLUSHED LUMENS

I've found a way to teach my patient with a multiple-lumen central venous catheter how to ensure that he's flushed all the lumens.

After we prepare the correct number of flushes, the patient and I decide how to refer to the flushing sequence of the lumens, such as left to right or shortest to longest. If the patient loses track of which lumens he flushed, he can count the flushes he has left and immediately know which lumen to flush next.

KINK ELIMINATOR

Here's what I do to prevent a multiple-lumen catheter from kinking: I cut a straw to the desired length, then split it lengthwise. I place the tubing in the straw, then lightly tape over the split to keep the straw in place. Because the straw encases the tubing, it prevents kinks. This procedure also works well on feeding tubes.

QUICK FIX FOR A CRACKED PORT

Here's a way to fix temporarily a cracked side port on a central venous line introducer: Insert a 14-gauge over-the-needle catheter into the lumen and remove the needle. This will prevent air from entering the vessel, fluid from leaking out, and the lumen from clotting. Now you can use the port until you have the opportunity to change it.

PICC POINTER

Helpful insertion reminder: The two basilic veins are the preferred sites for peripherally inserted central catheter (PICC) insertion. Why? They are straighter than the cephalic vein and they widen gradually as they become axillary veins.

PICC PROTECTOR

I've discovered a way to help my patients keep a peripherally inserted central catheter (PICC) dry while taking a shower.

I take a long plastic bag used to hold disposable cups and cut off both ends of the bag to fit my patient's arm, have the patient slide his arm into the bag, and wrap tape around the plastic bag at both ends. This technique avoids taping the patient's skin.

NUMBING A PORT SITE

A patient with an implanted port may have some pain when you insert a needle into the port. So I put ice chips over the port site for a short time to numb the area. Then the patient feels less discomfort.

VAP ADVICE #1

Always check for correct needle placement when accessing a venous access port (VAP). You can do this by aspirating for a blood return. If you can't obtain a blood return, the catheter leading from the port may be lodged against the vessel wall.

VAP ADVICE #2

If you are unable to obtain a blood return after entering a venous access port (VAP), the catheter may be lodged against the vessel wall. To free it, ask the patient to try the following:
• Raise his arms.
• Perform Valsalva's maneuver.
• Change position.

If you are unsuccessful in freeing the catheter, notify the doctor; a fibrin sleeve may have formed on the distal end of the catheter.

Home blood transfusions

PREPARATION CHECKLIST
Don't administer a blood transfusion to a home care patient until you're sure the following conditions have been met:
• The patient has signed an informed consent.
• The patient's hemoglobin is below 10 mg/dl.
• The patient's medical diagnosis is nonacute.
• The patient is alert, cooperative, and able to respond to body symptoms.
• A responsible adult is present (in addition to the patient and the nurse).
• The transfusion requires no more than 3 units in a 24-hour period.
• Local emergency medical personnel are available if needed.

TEMP FOR TRANSPORT
The proper temperature for transporting blood is between 33.8° and 50° F (1° and 10° C); for platelets, it's between 68° and 75° F (20° and 24° C).

HOME MONITORING GUIDELINES
I tell my patients receiving home blood transfusions and their caregivers to be on the lookout for the following signs, and to call me or their doctor right away if any appear:
• rash or hives within the next 24 hours
• pain or bleeding at or near the infusion site
• red or brown urine appearing during the next 24 hours
• pinpoint or larger bruises appearing during the first week
• shortness of breath within the next 24 to 72 hours
• fever or shaking chills within the next 4 weeks.

TRANSFUSION TIP
The flush solution of choice for blood transfusions is 0.9% sodium chloride. Other solutions can cause problems. For

example, dextrose solutions cause red blood cells to clump, swell, and hemolyze; lactated Ringer's solution contains calcium, which can counteract the anticoagulant used in the blood bag.

Parenteral nutrition

A WARNING ABOUT WARMING

Warning: Never heat a parenteral feeding solution in a microwave oven; nutrients in the solution may decompose, and the glucose may caramelize.

Instead, try this easy warming method (I recommend it to my patients and their family members): Remove the solution from the refrigerator about an hour before it's needed, place it on a countertop, and leave it to warm to room temperature.

OVERCOME OVERFILL

If you, your patient, or the patient's caregiver accidently overfill the drip chamber with parenteral nutrition solution, do the following:

Invert the container and squeeze some of the solution back from the drip chamber into the solution container.

10

Procedures

Contents

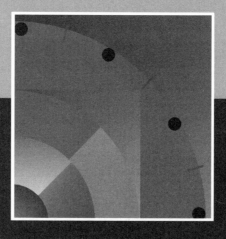

Contributors

The following nurses contributed tips and timesavers for this chapter:

Dee Adinaro, RN, MSN

Sheryl Stone Clay, RN, BSN

Irene Duquette, RN

Nina S. Ehle, RN

Trudy Fremont, RN, CFLE, MS

Patricia Maskell, RN, BSN

Mary J. O'Donnell, RN

D. Peters, RN

Elaine A. Peterson, RN

Cheryl Reich, RN

Kathy Scheeve, RN

Kay B. Stewart, RN, CS, MSN

Kathy Tweed, LPN

Personal care

CUSTOM CLOTHING

Here's a fast way to fashion a sleep shirt that's easy for patients to take on and off:

Buy an oversized, long- or short-sleeved T-shirt; then cut the shirt along the center back, leaving the neck band intact. Hem the cut edges—voilà—the shirt is ready to wear. You don't need to make back ties; the neck band will keep everything in place.

If your patient needs a bed jacket, create one from an oversized flannel shirt using the same technique.

ONE-ARMED BATHING

I always recommend that patients with an immobilized arm or hand use a sponge, not a washcloth, for personal grooming. A sponge is easy to handle, fits nicely into your patient's hand, is easy to wring (or squeeze) out, and doesn't require folding.

What's more, a sponge makes an effective exercise tool for a patient with arthritis; squeezing it helps loosen up stiff joints.

DENTURE LANDING PAD

Before you brush or rinse a patient's dentures, put a towel in the sink. That way, the dentures won't break if you drop them.

HASSLE-FREE SHAMPOO

I've discovered an effective way to wash an arthritic patient's hair without getting shampoo and water in her eyes or ears. This is what I do:

First, I cut the top out of a plastic shower cap. Then, I put the cap on my patient's head, placing the plastic rim above her ears and eyebrows, and pull her hair through the newly

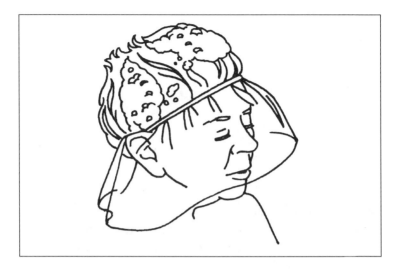

created opening. Next, I flip down the remaining cap to protect her face.

It's a relief not to have to ask my patient to tilt her head back (a movement that's painful for her). And I know she won't be getting water in her eyes and ears.

MOUTH CARE TECHNIQUE

Giving mouth care to a patient who must lie flat in bed isn't easy—especially the rinsing and spitting. But here's a way to avoid the mess:

After the patient's teeth are brushed, offer him mouthwash or water through a straw. Then, have him use the same straw to expel the mouthwash or water into an emesis basin.

Although using a straw may be a bit awkward at first, patients usually master it quickly and become proficient in the ins and outs of rinsing and spitting with straws.

REMOVING ENCRUSTATIONS

I provide home care for a patient with such stubborn encrustations on his toes and nails that not even a vigorous soap-and-water scrub will remove them. My solution: A single application of a lemon-glycerine swab. This will gently remove the debris without causing discomfort or tissue damage.

Heat and cold therapy

ICE ADVICE
When filling an ice bag for a patient, I use small chips of ice. This makes the bag flexible and easy to mold to the patient's body.

PUNCTURE PREVENTION
Never secure an ice bag or any other cooling device with pins; an accidental puncture may allow icy fluid to leak out and burn the patient's skin.

COOL COMFORT
I've discovered an excellent material for protecting a patient's skin when applying nonsterile cold therapy: a thin sheet of foam. Traditional washcloth or pillowcase barriers become too cold and wet; the patient cannot tolerate them long enough for treatment to be effective. A foam pad, however, keeps the patient dry and comfortable (condensation rolls off the foam to padding placed under the treatment area). The patient should be able to tolerate at least 15 minutes of treatment. This technique works well for cold applications to the pelvis, eye, and facial areas.

SAVE WHILE YOU SOAK
Here's how one of my patients minimizes the cost of soaking his feet in a prescribed (but nonsterile) soaking solution:

The patient pours the solution into a clean plastic bag and puts his foot into the bag. Then, he loosely fastens the bag with a wide strip of cloth. He places the bagged foot into a bucket of warm water.

The water not only warms the solution, but also causes it to rise in the bag to the level of the water in the bucket. This way,

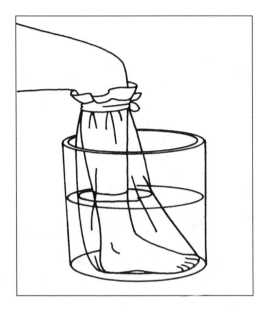

the patient uses less solution to cover his foot and saves money. This method works for soaking a hand as well.

Elimination

URINAL CLEANER
When providing home care, I use denture cleaner to remove sediment, stains, and odor from urinals. I simply pour hot water into the urinal and then add 1 tablet of denture cleaner (such as Polident) daily.

STOMA ODOR STOPPER
In addition to using vinegar to clear his stoma, your patient can eliminate embarrassing urinary stoma odor by drinking cranberry juice or apple juice and taking vitamin C tablets. These measures acidify urine and reduce odor.

KINK-PROOFING A CATHETER
Preventing kinks in indwelling catheter tubing is a daily challenge, especially when a patient is restless and twists and

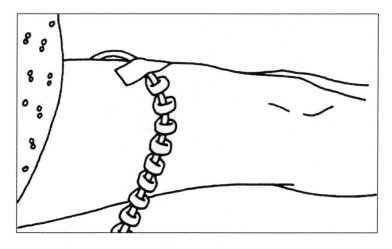

turns a lot. If the tubing kinks, the patient can develop urinary reflux, leakage, or even a urinary tract infection. To stop
kinking, wrap a coil-type phone cord around the tubing.
Even if the patient twists and turns, the tubing won't kink.

ENEMA ADMINISTRATION ADVICE
If the flow stops when administering an enema, the tubing
may be compressed against the rectal wall or clogged with
feces. To free the tubing without stimulating defecation, gently turn it slightly. If the tubing is clogged, withdraw it, flush
with solution, and then reinsert it.

KEEPING THE LID UP
Do you find that a commode lid has a penchant for slam-
ming shut just as you lower your patient onto the seat? Here's
a good way to keep the lid up.

Get a Velcro book latch (used to hold large chart pages
open) that has two parts: a long tab (A) and a circle (B).
Attach the adhesive side of B to the underside of the commode lid. Then attach the adhesive side of A to the commode
frame with one end of the tab hanging down. (The tab's
Velcro side should face away from the commode.)

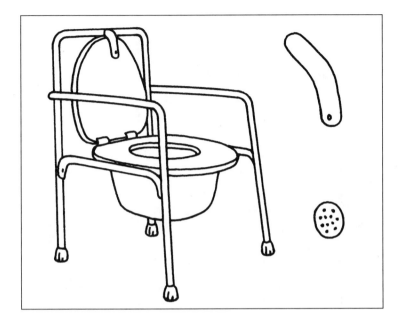

Before you help the patient onto the commode, bring tab A up over the lid and secure it to circle B on the lid. The lid will remain raised until you undo the latch.

EASING ENEMA INSERTION
The following technique helps me insert enema tubing with minimal discomfort to the patient:

Before inserting the tubing, I touch the patient's anal sphincter with the tip of the tube to stimulate contraction. Then, as the sphincter relaxes, I tell the patient to breathe deeply through the mouth while I gently advance the tube.

OSTOMY ADVICE
Never apply ostomy paste where it could block drainage.

OSTOMY WAFERS: PREVENTING PERSPIRATION
Tell your ostomy patient to wipe his skin with a 5-day deodorant pad before applying an ostomy wafer. This will help control perspiration, thereby preventing the wafer from

loosening. He'll also save money because he won't need to change his appliance as often.

PREVENTING ILEOSTOMY BLOCKAGE

In my years of home care practice, I've found that certain foods are more likely to block an ileostomy than others. Foods more likely to cause blockage include popcorn, peanuts, high-cellulose vegetables, round steak, coconut, and string beans. Some patients may need to avoid these foods altogether. I encourage all ileostomy patient's I care for to chew their food thoroughly and take frequent, small sips of liquid during meals.

MEASURING RESIDUAL URINE

Seeking to measure residual urine in the bladder? Make sure the patient voids immediately before you insert the catheter.

OVERCOMING CATHETER RESISTANCE

Here's a technique I use when I'm advancing a catheter into a male patient and the catheter meets resistance:

I gently pull on the penis so the glans points toward the umbilicus. Pulling straightens the urethra, thereby helping to overcome resistance.

TAPING TECHNIQUE

A patient with catheter tubing taped to his thigh or abdomen may develop skin sensitivity and irritation. To minimize irritation, I alternate sides each time I retape the tubing.

SKIN PROTECTION: SOCK IT TO ME

A patient with a urinary leg bag may develop skin rashes and excoriation, especially in warm weather. Here's how I make him more comfortable.

I cut off the foot of a tube sock and pull the sock over the patient's knee to midthigh; I make sure the sock isn't too tight. The bag rests against the sock—which protects the patient's skin—and is secured with the leg strap. The sock is easy to keep clean, and it absorbs perspiration.

Gastrointestinal therapy

STIFF YET FLEXIBLE
Having inserted many nasogastric tubes, I learned how to adjust the stiffness to make insertion easier:

To stiffen a tube, I place it in a tray of ice chips; to relax one, I place it in warm water for a few minutes.

FEEDING WITH A SYRINGE
The following techniques help prevent air from entering a patient's stomach when administering an intermittent bolus tube feeding:

During administration, never empty the syringe completely. Administer the feeding slowly, usually 200 to 350 ml over 10 to 15 minutes, depending on the patient's tolerance and the doctor's order.

TUBE LENGTH MEMORY AID
Use this mnemonic to remember how to determine the appropriate length for a nasogastric tube: NEX. Interpretation: Measure from the tip of the Nose to the Earlobe to the Xiphoid process.

TO A TEE
Surgical patients discharged with a long-term or permanent feeding tube, which must be clamped between feedings to prevent backflow, sometimes lose the clamp and are unable to find a replacement. A plastic or wooden golf tee is a readily available substitute that fits perfectly into the end of a nasogastric tube.

COOL FOOD IN HOT WEATHER
During the hot summer months, a home care patient's enteral feeding bag may not stay cool enough. If that's a problem,

slip the feeding bag and a frozen cold pack (the kind used in coolers for picnics) into a plastic storage bag. Punch a hole in the storage bag, about 2" (5 cm) up, for the feeding tube. Then wrap the bag in a towel to absorb condensation.

This will reduce the risk of bacterial growth in the enteral food.

CLEANING WITH COLA

When a feeding tube becomes clogged with formula, unclog it with diet cola. Get a doctor's order first; then flush the feeding tube with 1 oz (30 ml) of cola. Clamp the tube for 15 minutes. The cola will dissolve the formula and unclog the tube.

CLEANING WITH CRANBERRY JUICE

Small-diameter enteral feeding tubes often get clogged from the feeding formula residue. To prevent this residue buildup, we flush the tubes every 4 hours (and each time the feeding is interrupted or discontinued) with ⅔ oz (20 ml) of cranberry juice, followed by ⅓ oz (10 ml) of water.

The acidic cranberry juice breaks up the formula's residue, and the water rinses away the juice, preventing sugar from crystallizing in the tube.

VEGETABLE-OILED SYRINGE

Many of my home care patients who receive frequent gastrostomy tube feedings find that the plungers of their 60-ml syringes become stiff and difficult to slide into the barrel of the syringe. To make the syringes easier to insert, I advise my patients to dip the tip of the plunger in vegetable oil before each feeding. Then the plunger will slide with ease.

Skin care

MONEY-SAVING RELIEF FOR ITCHY SKIN

Oatmeal-based bath packets are effective in relieving pruritus, but they're expensive. My alternative:

I place ½ to ¾ cup (about 120 to 180 ml) of quick-cooking raw oatmeal in a cotton sock. Then I saturate and wring out the sock under the bathtub spout as the tub is filling with water. The oatmeal sock makes the water as soothing as a bath packet would, at a much lower price.

THE SQUEEZE TEST

When it comes to foam used to protect my patient from pressure areas, how thick is thick enough? To find out, I use my favorite test: the squeeze test. I squeeze the foam between my fingers. If I can feel my fingers through the foam, I need a thicker piece. Usually about 1½" (3.8 cm) thickness suffices. The denser the foam, the better the reduction of pressure.

THROW IN THE TOWEL

This tip can save an incontinent patient and his family hundreds of dollars a year.

Families often purchase disposable blue pads to place under the patient when he or she rests in bed or sits on upholstered furniture. These pads cost about $.50 each and a patient may use several a day.

A less expensive alternative: a towel or soft cloth placed over a large trash bag. The fabric will absorb wetness; the plastic bag will contain it. And the family can simply wash the towel when it's soiled.

ANTACID DABS

Dabbing antacid on periostomal skin may ease irritation caused by fluid leaks or pouches applied to damp skin. But it shouldn't be used routinely or prophylactically because it may interfere with the skin's normal pH. Try to determine the source of the irritation and correct it.

Wound care

DRESSING FOR DEEP WOUNDS

When one of my patients has a deep wound with copious drainage, I use an exudate absorber, such as calcium alginate, copolymer starch, or dextranomer beads. The dressing will soak up drainage and fill dead space in the wound cavity. It will even fill sinus tracts. However, if the wound has sinus tracts, make sure that the dressing can be removed with irrigation.

HOMEMADE SOLUTION GUIDELINES

Before making any solution in your patient's home, boil the water for 20 minutes and let it cool. And use a lidded storage bottle or jar that has been sanitized in the dishwasher or in boiling water for 20 minutes.

HOMEMADE 0.9% SODIUM CHLORIDE SOLUTION

To make 0.9% sodium chloride solution, use 2 teaspoons table salt and 1 quart of boiled water. Measure the boiled water and pour it into a jar that has been sanitized in the dishwasher or in boiling water for 20 minutes. Add the table salt and mix well. Cover with a lid. For sterile procedures, prepare a new supply every day; for clean procedures, store the solution in the refrigerator for up to 1 week.

HOMEMADE ACETIC ACID SOLUTION

To make ¼ strength acetic acid solution, use 4 tablespoons white distilled vinegar and 5 cups of boiled water. Measure the boiled water and pour it into a jar that has been sanitized in the dishwasher or in boiling water for 20 minutes. Add the vinegar and mix well. Cover with a sterile lid and store in a cool place. This recipe makes about 1 quart of solution that is stable for approximately 1 week.

HOMEMADE DAKIN'S SOLUTION

To prepare Dakin's solution at home, use approximately 1⅔ ounces of household bleach and 1 quart of boiled water for a full-strength solution. Use approximately 1 ounce household solution and 1 quart of water for half strength. Pour the bleach into a jar that has been sanitized in the dishwasher or in boiling water for 20 minutes and add the boiled water. Cover with a sterile lid and store in a cool place. This recipe makes about 1 quart of solution that is stable for approximately 1 week.

TAKING OUT THE STING

Take the sting out of removing old dressings from a patient with hairy skin; use an acetone free adhesive solvent or baby oil to free the tape and lessen discomfort.

SEPARATION SOLUTION

Some dressings and wounds just won't part company. If your patient's dressing stubbornly adheres to the wound, try moistening the gauze with 0.9% sodium chloride solution.

TRANSPARENT DRESSING GUIDELINES

When is a transparent film dressing an appropriate choice? And when is it best avoided? Follow the guidelines below.

Use transparent film dressings:
• for partial-thickness wounds
• for stage II pressure ulcers
• for autolytic debridement on wounds that have dry necrosis
• as secondary dressings over wound packing material to protect it from moisture or invading organisms.

Do not use transparent film dressings for:
• deep wounds
• wounds with sinus tracts
• wounds with excessive drainage or fragile periwound tissue.

COLLECTING WOUND SPECIMENS

Need to collect specimens from an infected wound? Avoid collecting old exudate, which may be contaminated with resident bacteria, which is different from bacteria causing the infection. Rinse the wound with 0.9% sodium chloride solution, then take the specimens.

IMPROVISING MONTGOMERY STRAPS

Here's a quick and easy way to make Montgomery straps from hypoallergenic tape:

Cut four to six strips of tape long enough to extend about 6" (15 cm) beyond the edges of the wound. Take one strip and fold 2" to 3" (5 to 8 cm) back, sticky sides together, to form a nonadhesive tab.

Fold the tab lengthwise, then crosswise, and snip off a diagonal section of the folded corner. When the tab is unfolded, you'll have a diamond-shaped hole in the center of the tab.

Repeat these steps to make as many straps as needed.

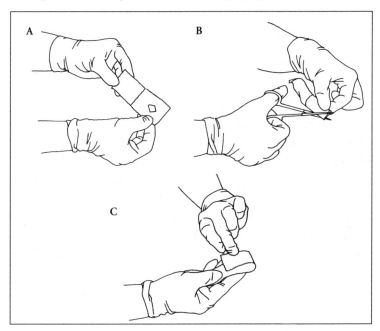

SPECIFYING WOUND SPECIMENS
When I take more than one specimen from the same infected wound, I number each sample. Then I document in my patient's chart and on the laboratory slips where each specimen came from. For example, # 1—upper left corner; #2—middle third of wound.

FROM THE INCISION OUTWARD
To decrease the risk of contaminating a wound, I always start cleaning at the incision and wipe outward.

Respiratory therapy

PREVENTING OXYGEN TOXICITY
Whenever I care for a patient on home oxygen therapy, I watch for early signs of oxygen toxicity. If I intervene promptly, I can save my patient a trip to the hospital. The signs I look for include:
• retrosternal distress
• difficulty breathing
• numbness, prickling, or tingling in the arms and legs
• lethargy or restlessness
• anorexia.

NASOPHARYNGEAL SUCTIONING
Inserting a catheter into the nose for nasopharyngeal suctioning requires a careful touch. My suggestion: Slightly rotate the catheter between your thumb and index finger to ease insertion.

OXYGEN THERAPY TIP
Here's a quick tip for securing an oxygen cannula. Don't attach it too tightly; excessive pressure may contribute to skin breakdown or occlusion of the nasal prongs.

OXYGEN THERAPY WHISTLE
If you hear a high-pitched whistling sound while your patient is receiving oxygen therapy, look for an obstruction such as pinched or closed tubing. The noise comes from pressure backing up in the humidifier and escaping through a positive pressure relief valve.

EASING ANXIETY
Many patients find a continuous positive-airway pressure (CPAP) mask uncomfortable and confining. Worse, it makes them feel anxious. To help relieve my patients' discomfort and enhance compliance, I provide thorough patient teaching and reassurance and assist patients to relax and breath normally.

PROTECTING THE EAR
An oxygen cannula may cause skin breakdown on top of a patient's ear. If so, clear the area and cut a sterile bandage lengthwise. Place the bandage over the ear and rest the can-

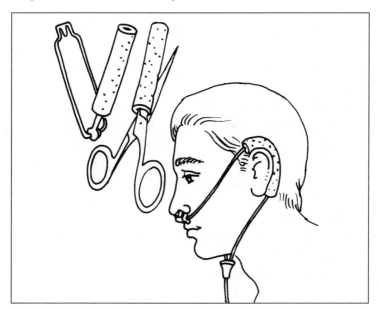

nula on the gauze portion. That should relieve the pressure.
Or you can use a foam curler: Slit it lengthwise and slide it
over the cannula at the ear.

Pain control

TENS ELECTRODE CARE
After removing the electrodes from a patient's skin at the end
of a transcutaneous electrical nerve stimulator (TENS) treatment, I clean the patient's skin with alcohol and clean the
electrodes with soap and water. Tip: To avoid damaging the
electrodes, do not soak them in alcohol.

PAIN MANAGEMENT
Home care patients have just as great a need for pain relief as
hospital patients. Keep in mind these factors which may
interfere with effective pain control therapy:
• misconceptions, such as believing patients exaggerate
reports of pain
• fear of narcotic addiction
• inadequate education of patients and family members
regarding pain control
• inconsistencies with pain assessment or documentation and
poor communication among health care providers
• patient noncompliance such as not taking a drug as scheduled because of adverse drug effects.

IMPORTANT LESSON
Over a decade of experience in home care nursing has taught
me one crucial fact about pain control: Pain is what the
patient says it is. In other words, pain is subjective and no
tests can measure it objectively. When providing nursing care,
believe the patient's report of pain.

11

Nursing Law

Contents

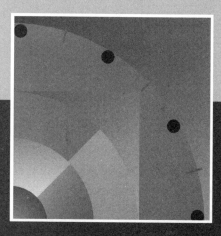

Contributors

The following nurses and attorneys provided tips and timesavers for this chapter:

Barbara E. Calfee, JD

Sr. Roberta Downey, RN

Ann Dodge, RN, ET

Donna Edelmann, RN

Ellen Thomas Eggland, RN, MN

Nancy B. Grane, RN, BS

Mary Hartz, RN, BSN

Patricia Iyer, RN, CNA, MSN

Roseanne M. Ottaggio, RN, CDE, MSN

Documentation

PICTURE POWER

To reduce Medicare denials for reimbursement of home nursing care, my colleagues and I use photographs to document a patient's need for wound care.

First, we obtain written permission from patients to photograph wounds that will need extensive—and costly—treatment. Then, we take two photos of the affected area, keeping a copy of one in the patient's chart. The originals are sent to Medicare with the patient's claim form. If necessary, we photograph the wound later to document healing.

BODY STAMP

When we chart information on a patient with a pressure sore, we use a black ink stamp showing the outline of the human body. Then we circle the location of the pressure sore; label it

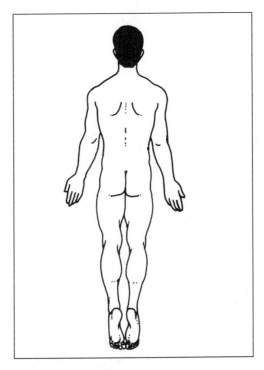

for size, stage, and drainage; and describe other significant characteristics (such as redness, edema, and odor). We use the stamp on progress notes, care plans, treatment forms, assessment forms, and discharge plans. This charting aid quickly communicates important information.

SKIN STAMP
Describing wounds and their treatment can be a time-consuming part of charting. I developed a skin documentation stamp to make the job easier. This stamp includes space for recording the location, size, and depth of the wound and for describing the tissue, drainage, and treatment. All I have to do is fill in the blanks.

HANDY RULER
When you need to assess and document wounds, your index finger can function as a tool for estimating wound size. Measure each section of your finger and remember its length. That way, you'll have a measuring aid that's always "handy."

REPORTING AN INCIDENT
When an incident occurs, do you ever wonder if you're documenting the incident adequately? Here are some tips to help you:
• Only the person who witnessed the incident or first discovered it should file an incident report, and only that person should sign it. Anyone else with firsthand knowledge should file a separate report. Check your agency's policy and procedure manuals for incidents that should be reported and the forms and procedures to use.
• Record the details in objective terms, describing exactly— and only—what you saw or heard. For example: "Found patient on floor beside bed" not "Patient fell from bed."
• Describe what you did at the scene, such as helping the patient back to bed, and your assessment findings. Also note any instructions you gave to the patient—for example, telling

her to call a caregiver for help if she wants to get out of bed again.
• Document the time of the incident, the name of the doctor you notified, and the time you notified him. Also notify your manager and have her review the form.
• Incident reports should be retained by the agency administrators, not included in the patient's chart.
• Chart clinical details related to the incident (for example, assessment findings and treatments). Just make sure the progress notes and incident report are consistent with each other.

LEGALLY-SAFE ABBREVIATIONS

To prevent ambiguity that could lead to treatment errors, remember these three cardinal rules about using abbreviations.
1. *Use only those abbreviations approved by your agency.*
Remember: Approved abbreviations differ from agency to agency, so you'll need to check the list used in your agency.
2. *Write legibly.* Even approved abbreviations can be misunderstood if they're not written clearly. And anything that's illegible to a staff member will surely stump a jury in a malpractice suit.
3. *Always explain abbreviations that can have more than one meaning.* Write out the potentially confusing term or word on first reference, followed by the approved abbreviation in parentheses.

DETAILS, DETAILS

To avoid "broad-brushing" your narrative notes, always remember to include the following:
• specific information, including distances, quantities, time frames, and pertinent patient comments
• assessment findings that substantiate your interventions. Check that your assessment findings don't contradict your interventions. For example, it wouldn't seem appropriate to

include an intervention for raising side rails for a patient who's oriented to person, place, and time and has good balance, a steady gait, stable vital signs, and no dizziness.
• any specific precautions that other nurses participating in the patient's care should take.

TRACHEOSTOMY CARE: FLOW OF FACTS

To save charting time when caring for a tracheostomy patient, my coleagues and I have developed an interdisciplinary tracheostomy flow sheet. In 8 one-line entries, we can document the type and amount of secretions and aspirate, frequency of suctioning and basic care, and presence of a cough.

The flow sheet not only saves time, but also organizes information about the patient's care. Other service providers can glance at the sheet for a quick assessment of the patient's condition and care during the previous 24 hours.

PHONE ORDER FOLLOW-THROUGH

Almost every home care nurse faces this situation at some point: Your patient needs treatment right away and you have no choice but to obtain a telephone order. Remember to carefully follow your agency's policy for documenting the telephone order. Generally, you'll follow this procedure:
• Repeat the order, using the patient's name. For example, you'd say, "Doctor, you're ordering oxygen, 4 liters per minute, by nasal cannula and 40 mg Lasix P.O daily for William Perry, correct?"
• Record the order on the doctor's order sheet as soon as possible. First, note the date and time; then write the order verbatim. On the next line, write "t.o." for telephone order. Then, write the doctor's name and sign your name.
• Draw lines through any blank spaces in the order.
• Make sure the doctor countersigns the order within the time limits set by your agency's policy. Without his signature, you may be held liable for practicing medicine without a license.

ADVICE: BE PRECISE
When you document, you must make sure other caregivers know *exactly* what you mean—by giving precise times, amounts, sizes, and other characteristics. To describe dimension, you can use examples, such as "raised, pea-size cyst." Be concise but clear; reread your notes to make sure they're accurate. And always use correct medical terms and abbreviations approved by your facility; double-check if you're not sure.

CHARTING WITH UNCLE SAM IN MIND
To ensure your patient qualifies for Medicare coverage, make sure your documentation substantiates the following:
• The patient meets Medicare coverage requirements.
• The doctor ordered the services.
• You provided the services as ordered.
• The services were reasonable and necessary.
• You supervised staff members as needed.

MEETING THE CHARTING CHALLENGE
In home care nursing, thoroughness and accuracy in charting are essential to ensuring continuity of care and to obtaining reimbursement. In fact, in no other health care setting are you as responsible for ensuring reimbursement payments as you are in the home health setting. Here's a quick rundown of the most essential guidelines:
• Use specific terms; don't be vague. For example, accurately list the patient's vital signs; never just say, "stable" or, "within normal limits."
• Document the patient's condition, all nursing interventions, instructions provided to the patient and family, and the patient's and family's understanding of interventions and instructions.
• Document coordination among all disciplines providing care through your agency.
• Document the plan for follow-up care or discharge.

PSYCHOSOCIAL STATUS CHECKLIST
Here's a quick list of factors to include when documenting psychosocial status during the initial home visit:
• living conditions
• economic situation
• culture
• availability of caregiver
• primary language (including the caregiver's primary language)
• ability and motivation to learn (also note the caregiver's ability and motivation to learn)
• coping styles
• support systems
• access to transportation.

MEDICAL HISTORY CHECKLIST
Here's a quick set of guidelines for performing and documenting the medical history and physical exam during the initial home visit:
• Focus primarily on acute medical instabilities (especially factors that may influence homebound status). Document findings carefully.
• Assess functional limitations of the patient and caregiver, including mobility, dexterity, vision, hearing, and strength.
• Assess and document home safety needs.

DOCUMENTING MEDS
Here's how I fine-tune documentation of my patient's medication regimen:

During the first home visit, I ask the patient to show me everything he or she is taking, including over-the-counter drugs and health supplements, such as vitamins. Then, I carefully document each medication.

Because Medicare will provide reimbursement for teaching a patient about new medications (in certain instances, it will reimburse for teaching about previous or altered prescriptions), I make sure my plan of care reflects the status (new, old, or changed) of each prescription and over-the-counter medication.

GETTING THE HELP YOU NEED

With regard to writing orders for specific skilled and unskilled services, experience has taught me to provide plenty of details. First, I indicate the type of service to be provided, and then frequency of the service. Here's how I describe frequency:

I specify both the number of weeks for visits and the number of visits per week. The number of visits per week usually decreases as the patient gets better. To ensure the most appropriate level of care, I give a range of frequencies for visits. For example, SN 5-7 wk $\times$ 1, 3-5 wk $\times$ 4, 1-3 wk $\times$ 4, indicates that skilled nursing will be provided five to seven times a week for 1 week. The frequency will then decrease to three to five visits a week for 4 weeks, and go to one to three a week for the remaining 4 weeks of the certification period.

JUSTIFYING NEED

When my patient needs a specific service, I've learned to carefully justify this need in my documentation. For example, I document precisely why my patient or caregiver can't or won't learn to perform a skill or procedure. I identify the patient's or caregiver's knowledge deficits regarding new or changed medications, procedures, and diagnoses.

MEDICARE REIMBURSEMENT

I provide home care to an elderly patient who requires patient, repeated instruction to learn new self-care skills. I've had to be especially careful when documenting this situation. Medicare won't reimburse for repeated instruction—unless the patient (or his caregiver) states he forgot or is unsure of a specific instruction. If the caregiver is new, Medicare will provide reimbursement.

In your documentation, clearly state any change that took place to necessitate repeated instruction, for example, a new caregiver or a change in dosage. Refrain from using terms that suggest repetitive instruction, such as reinforced, reviewed, reinstructed, and reminded. Avoid using the word encourage; Medicare and other payers don't consider encouraging to be a "skilled service."

JUST THE FACTS
My agency emphasizes maintaining objectivity when documenting visits. Here's what I've learned through training and experience boiled down to three simple phrases:
• Write down only what you've seen or know.
• Don't speculate about what might be there or why.
• Elaborate, using objective data, on any abnormal assessment findings.

HOME CARE DOCUMENTATION MUST
Be certain to state in your documentation that the patient is housebound and provide the reason for this. Keep in mind that Medicare requires that a patient receiving skilled care in the home must be housebound, although some commercial insurers do not.

PEOPLE NOT PAPER
To prevent your patient from feeling neglected, do not spend a lot of time charting in his home. Consider completing your records while the patient sleeps or is otherwise occupied, back in your car, or back at the agency's office.

PATIENT PARTICIPATION
Whenever possible, use flow sheets and checklists to record vital signs, intake and output measurements, and nutritional data. Encourage the patient or home caregiver to fill out these forms when appropriate. Doing so involves the patient and family in the patient's progress and increases their feeling of control.

Patient rights

INFORMED CONSENT CHECKLIST

If you know a patient has not been informed about an upcoming treatment or procedure and you do nothing, you can be held legally responsible. Establish whether or not a patient has given "informed consent" by asking yourself these questions:

• Has the patient received a written explanation of the treatment?

• Has the patient received an oral explanation of treatment options and the risks associated with those options?

• Does the patient understand what he has read and heard?

• Has the patient provided written consent freely and without coercion?

If the answer to any of these questions is no, tell the responsible health care provider (usually the patient's doctor) immediately.

PROTECTING CONFIDENTIALITY

Who can see your patient's chart? In most cases you can't reveal confidential information—even to one of the patient's close relatives—without the patient's permission.

So don't release the chart to anyone who's not authorized, and don't give oral information about your patient to anyone, including visitors, police officers, or insurance investigators. If you're not sure how to handle a request for information, notify the doctor and refer the request to the appropriate agency administrator.

However, the law requires disclosure of confidential information in certain situations—for example, those involving child abuse, public health hazards, and criminal cases. Certain agencies, such as the Internal Revenue Service and public health departments, can also order disclosure of the information.

Who else might be authorized to see the chart? Here are a few guidelines:
• The patient may see his own chart, and so may health care workers directly involved in his care.
• The next of kin or the patient's legally authorized representative may seek information if the patient isn't competent.
• The agency may allow health care workers to review records for research, statistical evaluation, and education.

For details about rules and exceptions that apply in your state, check with your agency's legal representative.

REFUSAL OF CARE
How should you respond when your patient refuses care? First provide the patient with information. For example:
• Explain the purpose of the treatment or procedure as well as the risks and complications that accompany it.
• Tell the patient who is to perform the treatment or procedure.
• Describe alternative treatments or procedures.
• Tell the patient the risks in not having the treatment performed.

If your patient still refuses, notify your supervisor. Document the patient's refusal in your nurses' notes, being sure to describe the information you provided to him. You may also be required to ask the patient to sign a refusal of treatment form.

Minimizing legal risks

ADVANCE DIRECTIVES
During your initial home visit, determine whether your patient has an advance directive. Be aware of the Patient Self-Determination Act of 1991. It requires agencies receiving federal funds to inquire whether patients admitted to their services have advance directives, such as a living will or a power of attorney for health care.

If the patient has such a document, the agency must abide by its provisions. If there is no such directive, and the patient wants to complete one, the agency must provide guidance.

ADVOCACY ABOVE ALL
If your patient has an advance directive, how will it affect your nursing role? Keep your responsibility as the patient's advocate in mind. Inform the doctor that the patient has expressed his wishes for treatment in such a document. If you feel strongly about the patient's right to have his wishes followed, work with family members and colleagues to come up with a unified plan of care.

LIVING WILL DILEMMA
What happens when a patient executes a living will in one state and later becomes terminally ill in another state? The law of the state where the living will decision will be carried out prevails.

If your patient has an out-of-state living will, you may need to determine whether it matches the criteria under the laws of the state you're in. Consult with your agency's attorney or refer the problem to your administrator.

LEGAL DISTINCTIONS
Quick quiz: What's the difference between a durable power of attorney and a health care power of attorney? A durable power of attorney is a legal instrument that gives another person the power to make decisions about financial matters and other civil affairs. It does not convey the right to make medical decisions. A health care power of attorney gives another person the power to make medical decisions if the patient becomes incompetent or too ill to express such decisions.

AVOIDING A DEFAMATION CHARGE

How can you protect yourself from being sued for defamation?

• Always make sure that what you say and write is an absolute fact, not an opinion.

• Discuss confidential information only with those who have an official reason to know. Remember: Fact doesn't justify a breach of confidentiality.

• Never allege another's negligence in an incident or editorialize about how an incident happened; just give the facts.

• Never write a derogatory comment about a colleague in the medical record, even if you believe it's the truth.

• When documenting your assessment of a patient, include only the objective findings; don't offer assumptions.

• Report an impaired colleague in good faith only—for example, after documenting examples of suspicious behavior.

• If you give performance evaluations, justify all negative comments with examples that illustrate your point.

• Avoid using labels such as "hostile," "rude," "aggressive," "difficult," "combative," or "crazy" to describe people. Instead, describe their behavior; it will speak for itself.

DOCUMENTING A MEDICATION ERROR

If a medication error occurs, your documentation should be as objective as possible. Remember, you're recording the facts of your patient's care and treatment. You're *not* giving details about why the error occurred; leave that for the incident report. Your notes should include:

• name and dosage of the medication and the time it was given

• patient's response to the medication

• name of the doctor and the time you notified him

• any nursing interventions or medical treatment

• patient's response to treatment.

SUPERVISOR BEWARE

Are you supervising one or more home health aides? Then be aware that all home health aides under your supervision must be properly trained. Federal law mandates strict qualification criteria for home health care aides who have a significant role in direct, hands-on contact with patients. Under the law, an agency may not use any individual who is not a licensed health care professional, *unless* the individual has successfully completed a training and competency evaluation program that meets minimum federal standards and the individual is competent to provide the services assigned.

Appendices

Contents

Commonly abused street drugs

SUBSTANCE	SYMPTOMS

Stimulants

Cocaine
• *Street names:* coke, flake, snow, nose candy, crack (hardened form), rock
• *Routes:* swallowing, injection, sniffing, smoking
• *Dependence:* psychological
• *Duration of effect:* 15 minutes to 2 hours; with crack, quick, short high followed by down feeling
• *Medical uses:* anesthetic

• *Of use:* abdominal pain, alternating euphoria and fear, appetite and weight loss, confusion, sweating, dilated pupils, excitability, fever, fast breathing, insomnia, irritability, nausea and vomiting, pale or blue skin, strange behavior, breathing stoppage, seizures, muscle spasms, sight, sound, and smell hallucinations
• *Of withdrawal:* anxiety, depression, fatigue

Amphetamines
• *Street names:* for amphetamine sulfate—bennies, cartwheels, goofballs; for methamphetamine—speed, meth, crystal, crank; for dextroamphetamine sulfate—dexies, hearts, oranges, greenies
• *Routes:* swallowing, injection, sniffing
• *Dependence:* psychological
• *Duration of effect:* 1 to 4 hours
• *Medical uses:* hypermobility, sleeping sickness, weight control

• *Of use:* altered mental state (from confusion to paranoia), sweating, dilated pupils, dry mouth, exhaustion, hallucinations, strange behavior (with prolonged use), seizures, shallow breathing, fast heartbeat, tremors
• *Of withdrawal:* abdominal tenderness, apathy, depression, disorientation, irritability, long periods of sleep, muscle aches, suicide attempts (with sudden withdrawal)

Hallucinogens

Lysergic acid diethylamide (LSD)
• *Street names:* acid, hits, microdot, sugar lump, big D, yellow kimples
• *Routes:* swallowing
• *Dependence:* possibly psychological
• *Duration of effect:* 8 to 12 hours
• *Medical uses:* none

• *Of use:* abdominal cramps; irregular heartbeat; chills; loss of identity; lost touch with reality; sweating; diarrhea; distorted perception of sight, time, and space; dizziness; dry mouth; fever; hallucinations; feeling of importance; heightened sense of awareness; fast breathing; illusions; increased salivation; muscle aches; mystical experiences; nausea; palpitations; seizures; vomiting
• *Of withdrawal:* none

Phencyclidine
• *Street names:* PCP, hog, angel dust, peace pill, crystal superjoint, elephant tranquilizer, rocket fuel, black bag, getting wet
• *Routes:* swallowing, injection, smoking
• *Dependence:* possibly psychological
• *Duration of effect:* 30 minutes to several days
• *Medical uses:* veterinary anesthetic

• *Of use:* amnesia; blank stare; decreased awareness of surroundings; delusions; distorted body image; distorted sense of sight, hearing, and touch; drooling; euphoria; excitation; fever; shuffling gait; hallucinations; hyperactivity; individualized unpredictable effects; muscle rigidity; panic; poor perception of time and distance; recurrent coma; kidney failure; seizures; sudden behavioral changes; extremely fast heartbeat; violent behavior
• *Of withdrawal:* none

SUBSTANCE	SYMPTOMS

Drepressants

Alcohol
• *Found in:* beer, wine, distilled spirits, cough syrup, after-shave, and mouthwash
• *Route:* swallowing
• *Dependence:* physical, psychological
• *Duration of effect:* varies from person to person and according to the amount swallowed
• *Medical uses:* release nerves from adhesions (absolute ethyl alcohol), emergency reduction of uterine contractions, treatment of ethylene glycol and methanol poisoning

Of acute use: decreased inhibitions, euphoria followed by depression or hostility, impaired judgment, incoordination, slow breathing, slurred speech, unconsciousness, vomiting, coma
• *Of withdrawal:* delirium, hallucinations, tremors, seizures

Benzodiazepines
(Ativan, Centrax, Dalmane, Doral, Halcion, Klonapen, Librium, Paxipam, Restoril, Serax, Tranzene, Valium, Versed, Xanax)
• *Street names:* dolls, green and whites, yellow jackets
• *Routes:* swallowing, injection
• *Dependence:* physical, psychological
• *Duration of effect:* 4 to 8 hours
• *Medical uses:* anxiety, seizures, sedation, hypnosis

• *Of use:* uncoordination, drowsiness, increased self-confidence, relaxation, slurred speech
• *Of overdose:* confusion, drowsiness, slowed breathing, coma
• *Of withdrawal:* abdominal cramps, agitation, anxiety, sweating, extremely fast heartbeat, seizures, tremors, vomiting

Barbiturates
(Amytal, Seconal, Solfoton)
• *Street names:* for barbiturates—downers, barbs; for amobarbital—blue angels, blue devils; for phenobarbital—purple hearts, goofballs; for secobarbital—reds, red devils
• *Routes:* swallowing, injection
• *Dependence:* physical, psychological
• *Duration:* 1 to 16 hours
• *Medical uses:* anesthesia, seizures, sedation, hypnosis

• *Of use:* skin blisters, bluish skin, decreased consciousness (from confusion to coma), fever, flaccid muscles, uncontrollable eye movements, poor pupil reaction to light, slowed breathing
• *Of withdrawal:* agitation, anxiety, fever, insomnia, dizziness when rising from a sitting or lying position, extremely fast heartbeat, tremors
• *Of rapid withdrawal:* appetite and weight loss, apprehension, hallucinations, dizziness when rising from a sitting or lying position, seizures, tremors, weakness

(continued)

Commonly abused street drugs *(continued)*

SUBSTANCE	SYMPTOMS

Depressants *(continued)*

Narcotics
(codeine, heroin, morphine, Demerol, opium)
• *Street names:* for heroin—junk, horse, H, smack; for morphine—morph
• *Routes:* for codeine, Demerol, morphine—swallowing, injection, smoking; for heroin—swallowing, injection, inhalation, smoking; for opium—swallowing, smoking
• *Dependence:* physical, psychological
• *Duration of effect:* 3 to 6 hours
• *Medical uses:* for codeine— pain, cough; for heroin—none; for morphine, Demerol—pain; for opium—pain, diarrhea

• *Of use:* appetite and weight loss, irregular heartbeat, clammy skin, constipation, tiny pupils, decreased consciousness, detachment from reality, drowsiness, euphoria, impaired judgment, increased skin pigmentation over veins, lack of concern, lethargy, nausea, needle marks, seizures, shallow or slow breathing, skin sores, slurred speech, swollen or perforated nasal lining, varicose veins, inability to urinate, vomiting
• *Of withdrawal:* abdominal cramps, appetite and weight loss, chills, sweating, dilated pupils, irritability, nausea, panic, runny nose, tremors, watery eyes, yawning

Cannabinoids

Marijuana
• *Street names:* pot, grass, weed, Mary Jane, roach, reefer, joint, THC
• *Routes:* swallowing, smoking
• *Dependence:* psychological
• *Duration of effect:* 2 to 3 hours
• *Medical uses:* prevention of vomiting during chemotherapy

• *Of use:* agitation, lack of motivation, anxiety, asthma, bronchitis, reddened eyes, muscle weakness, delusions, distorted self-perception and sense of time, dry mouth, euphoria, hallucinations, impaired ability to understand, impaired short-term memory, mood changes, uncoordination, increased hunger, dizziness when rising from a sitting or lying position, paranoia, spontaneous laughter, extremely fast heartbeat, extremely vivid imagination
• *Of withdrawal:* chills, decreased appetite, weight loss, insomnia, irritability, nervousness, restlessness, tremors

Safety tips

To stay safe when providing home care, follow these safety tips:
• Be aware of your surroundings.
• Wear comfortable, unrestrictive clothing.
• Keep your automobile in good repair.
• Know the location of public phones or keep a cellular phone with you.
• Keep your automobile doors locked. Drive with the windows up.
• If you must make a visit after dark, phone ahead and ask the patient to turn on the outside lights and watch for you.
• Stay on main streets. Avoid shortcuts through alleys or vacant areas.
• Look like you are on a mission: Be confident and walk tall.
• Carry only minimal supplies, and keep your hands free.
• Keep your purse locked in the trunk. Don't carry it into homes.
• Wear minimal jewelry.
• If you suspect that a car is following you, drive to the nearest police station.
• If you suspect that someone is following you, walk into a business establishment.
• If an individual or group of people looks suspicious, cross to the other side of the street.
• When entering a home, ask if anyone else is at home.
• Carry out the visit close to an exit. If this is not possible, plan how to get out if a fire or personal safety threat occurs.
• Leave the home immediately if you feel threatened in any way.
• Always have your keys in your hand before leaving a home.
• If you ride a bus, know the bus schedule and have the fare ready.
• Use special care in stairwells and elevators.

Treatments for poisons

This chart presents the suggested treatments for several kinds of poisoning. To determine which treatment is appropriate, refer to pages 167 to 170.

Caution: This chart can't replace your call to a poison control center, doctor, or hospital emergency room. Follow your agency's protocol.

Suggested treatment

1 Small amounts of this substance aren't poisonous, so no treatment is necessary.

2 Make the victim vomit. Give ipecac syrup in the following dosages:
• *If the victim is under age 1:*
2 teaspoons followed by at least two glasses of water.
• *If the victim is age 1 or older:*
1 or 2 tablespoons followed by at least two glasses of water.
• *If the person is unconscious or having a seizure:* don't make him or her vomit. Call the poison control center, doctor, or emergency room for instructions.

3 Dilute or neutralize the poison with water or milk. Don't make the person vomit. Call the poison control center, doctor, or emergency room.

4 Dilute or neutralize the poison with water or milk. Don't make the person vomit. The substance may burn the mouth and throat. Call the poison control center, doctor, or emergency room.

5 Immediately rinse skin thoroughly with running water. Continue for at least 15 minutes. Call the poison control center, doctor, or emergency room for help.

6 Immediately rinse eyes with running water. Continue for 15 to 20 minutes. Call the poison control center, doctor, or emergency room for further instructions.

7 Get the person to fresh air immediately; start artificial respiration if necessary. Call the poison control center, doctor, or emergency room for further instructions.

8 Call the poison control center, doctor, or emergency room before attempting any first-aid treatment. Always follow your agency's policy.

A

acetaminophen, 2
acetone, 8
acids
    eye contamination, 6
    inhalation (if mixed with
        bleach), 7
    skin contamination, 5
    swallowing, 4
aerosols
    eye contamination, 6
    inhalation, 7
after-shave lotions
    less than ½ oz (15 ml), 1
    more than ½ oz (15 ml), 8
airplane glue, 8
alcohol
    eye contamination, 6
swallowing (large quantities;
    methanol, any amount), 8
alkalies
    eye contamination, 6
    inhalation, 7
    skin contamination, 5
    swallowing, 4
ammonia
    eye contamination, 6
    inhalation, 7
    swallowing, 8
amphetamines, 2
analgesics, 8
aniline dyes
    inhalation, 7
    skin contamination, 5
    swallowing, 8
antacids, 1

antibiotics
    less than 2 to 3 times total
        daily dose, 1
    more than 3 times total daily
        dose, 2
antidepressant drugs, 8
antifreeze (ethylene glycol)
    eye contamination, 6
    swallowing, 8
antihistamines, 2
antiseptics, 2
ant trap, 8
aquarium products, 8
arsenic, 8
aspirin, 2

B

baby oil, 1
ball-point pen ink (*see* inks)
barbiturates, 8
batteries
    dry cell (flashlight), 8
    mercury (hearing aid), 8
    wet cell (automobile), 4
benzene
    inhalation, 7
    skin contamination, 5
    swallowing, 8
birth control pills, 8
bleaches
    eye contamination, 6
    inhalation (when mixed with
        acids or alkalies), 7
    swallowing (liquid), 1
    swallowing (solid), 4
boric acid, 2
bromides, 2
bubble bath, 1

The number after each substance refers to the appropriate treatment described on page 166.

Treatments for poisons

C
camphor, 8
candles, 1
caps for cap pistols
   less than one roll, 1
   more than one roll, 8
carbon monoxide, 7
carbon tetrachloride
   inhalation, 7
   skin contamination, 5
   swallowing, 2
chalk, 1
chlorine bleach (*see* bleaches)
cigarettes
   swallowing (less than one), 1
   swallowing (one or more), 2
clay, 1
cleaning fluids, 8
cleanser (household), 8
Clinitest tablets, 4
cocaine, 8
codeine, 8
cold remedies, 8
cologne
   less than ½ oz (15 ml), 1
   more than ½ oz (15 ml), 2
corn removers, 4
cosmetics *(see specific type)*
cough medicines, 8
crayons
   children's, 1
   others, 8
cyanide, 8

D
dehumidifying packets, 1
denture adhesives, 1
denture cleansers, 4
deodorants, 1
deodorizer cakes, 8

deodorizers, room, 8
desiccants, 8
detergents
   dishwasher and phosphate-
      free, 4
   liquid/powder (general), 1
dextromethorphan hydrobro-
      mide, 2
diaper rash ointment, 1
dishwasher detergents (*see*
   detergents)
disinfectants, 3
drain cleaners (*see* lye)
dyes
   aniline (*see* aniline dyes)
   others, 8

E
epoxy glue, 8
epsom salts, 2
ethylene glycol (*see* antifreeze)
eye makeup, 1

F
fabric softeners, 2
fertilizers, 8
fishbowl products, 8
furniture polish, 8

G
gas (natural), 7
gasoline, 8
glue, 8

H
hair dyes
   eye contamination, 6
   skin contamination, 5
   swallowing, 8

hallucinogens, 8
hand cream, 1
hand lotions, 1
herbicides, 8
heroin, 8
hormones, 8
hydrochloric acid (*see* acids)

I
inks
   ball-point pen, 1
   indelible, 2
   laundry marking, 2
   printer's, 8
insecticides
   skin contamination, 5
   swallowing, 8
iodine, 8
iron, 8

K
kerosene, 8

L
laxatives, 2
lighter fluid, 8
liniments, 8
lipstick, 1
lye
   eye contamination, 6
   inhalation (if mixed with
      bleach), 7
   skin contamination, 5
   swallowing, 4

M
makeup, 1
markers (indelible), 1
   indelible, 2
   water soluble, 1

matches
   less than 12 wood or 20
      paper, 1
   more than 12 wood or 20
      paper, 8
Mercurochrome, 8
mercury
   metallic (thermometer), 8
   salts, 2
Merthiolate, 8
metal cleaners, 8
methyl alcohol, 8
methyl salicylate, 2
mineral oil, 1
model cement, 8
modeling clay, 1
morphine, 8
mothballs, 2

N
nail polish, 8
nail polish remover
   less than ½ oz (15 ml), 8
   more than ½ oz (15 ml), 2
narcotics, 8
nicotine (*see* cigarettes)

O
oil of wintergreen, 2
oven cleaner (*see* lye)

P
paint, 8
paint chips, 8
paint thinner, 8
pencils, 1
perfume (*see* cologne)
permanent wave solution
   eye contamination, 6
   swallowing, 4

The number after each substance refers to the appropriate treatment described on page 166.

Treatments for poisons

The number after each substance refers to the appropriate treatment described on page 166.

Tips for Good Samaritans

As a home care nurse, you face an increased likelihood of encountering a motor vehicle accident or similar emergency when traveling between assignments. Here are some steps to follow to reduce your malpractice risk should you choose to provide assistance.

• Always observe professional standards of nursing care, regardless of the setting.

• Care for the accident victim in the vehicle if you can do so safely.

• Move the victim only if he's in danger and if his condition allows. Avoid moving him needlessly. Remember every accident victim is presumed to have a cervical spine injury until proven otherwise, so immobilize his cervical spine prior to moving him.

• Keep his airway open.

• Administer cardiopulmonary resuscitation if necessary.

• Stop his bleeding.

• Determine his level of consciousness.

• Keep him warm.

• Ask the victim if he feels pain. If he does, assess the location, duration, and intensity of his pain.

• Allow only skilled personnel to attend or treat the victim.

• Stay at the scene until skilled emergency personnel arrive to assume responsibility for the care of the victim.

• Provide emergency personnel with information regarding the victim's condition and any treatment you administered.

• Guard the victim's personal property. Release it only to the police or members of his family.

• Avoid speculation about who or what caused the accident.

• Always maintain your personal safety.

Community resources

**Alcoholics Anonymous
World Services**
475 Riverside Dr.
New York, NY 10163
(212) 870-3400

**Alexander Graham Bell
Association for the Deaf**
3417 Volta Pl., N.W.
Washington DC 20007
(202) 337-5220

Alzheimer's Association
919 North Michigan Ave.,
Suite 1000
Chicago, IL 60611-1676
(800) 272-3900

American Cancer Society
1599 Clifton Rd., N.E.
Atlanta, GA 30329
(800) 227-2345

**American Diabetes
Association**
1660 Duke St.
Alexandria, VA 22314
(800) 342-2383

**American Foundation for
the Blind**
11 Penn Pl., Suite 300
New York, NY 10011
(800) 232-5463

American Kidney Fund
6110 Executive Boulevard,
Suite 1010
Rockville, MD 20852-3903
(800) 638-8299

American Liver Foundation
1425 Pompton Ave.
Cedar Grove, NJ 07009
(800) 223-0179

American Lung Association
1740 Broadway
New York, NY 10019-4374
(800) LUNG-USA
(800-586-4872)

**American Parkinson
Disease Association**
60 Bay St., Suite 401
Staten Island, NY 10301
(718) 981-8001

American Red Cross
8111 Gatehouse Rd.
Falls Church, VA 22042
(202) 737-8300

Arthritis Foundation
1314 Spring St., N.W.
Atlanta, GA 30309
(800) 283-7800

Centers for Disease Control and Prevention
1600 Clifton Rd., N.E.
Atlanta, GA 30333
(404) 639-3311

Crohn's and Colitis Foundation of America
386 Park Ave. South
New York, NY 10016-7374
(800) 343-3637

Epilepsy Foundation of America
4351 Garden City Dr.,
Suite 406
Landover, MD 20785
(301) 459-3700

Glaucoma Research Foundation
490 Post St., Suite 830
San Francisco, CA 94102
(800) 826-6693

Juvenile Diabetes Foundation International
432 Park Ave. South
New York, NY 10016-8013
(800) 223-1138

La Leche League International
1400 North Meacham Rd.
P.O. Box 4079
Schaumburg, IL 60168-4079
(800) 525-3243

March of Dimes Birth Defects Foundation
1275 Mamaroneck Ave.
White Plains, NY 10605
(914) 428-7100

Mended Hearts
7272 Greenville Ave.
Dallas, TX 75231
(214) 706-1442

Narcotics Anonymous
P.O. Box 9999
Van Nuys, CA 91409
(818) 780-3951

National Association for Continence
P.O. Box 8310
Spartanburg, SC 29305-8310
(800) BLADDER
(800) 252-3337

National Associations of Area Agencies on Aging
1112 16th St., N.W.,
Suite 100
Washington, DC 20036
(202) 296-8130

National Council on Alcoholism and Drug Dependence
12 West 21 St.
New York, NY 10010
(212) 206-6770

Community resources

National Down Syndrome Society
666 Broadway
New York, NY 10012
(800) 221-4602

National Easter Seal Society
230 West Monroe St.
Chicago, IL 60606
(312) 726-6200

National Mental Health Association
1021 Prince St.
Alexandria, VA 22314-2971
(800) 969-6642

National Multiple Sclerosis Society
733 Third Ave.
New York, NY 10017
(800) FIGHT MS
(800) 344-4867

National Osteoporosis Foundation
1150 17th St., N.W.,
Suite 500
Washington, DC 20036
(800) 223-9994

United Ostomy Association
36 Executive Park, Suite 120
Irvine, CA 92714
(800) 826-0826

Selected references

The Clinical Answer Book. Springhouse, Pa.: Springhouse Corp., 1996.

Grossman, D. "Cultural Dimensions in Home Health Care Nursing," *AJN* 96(7):33-36, 1996.

Kendra, M.A. et al. "Safety Concerns Affecting Delivery of Home Health Care," *Public Health Nurse* 13(2):83-89, April 1996.

Maklebust, J. and Sieggreen, M. *Pressure Ulcers: Guidelines for Prevention and Nursing Management,* 2nd ed. Springhouse, Pa.: Springhouse Corp., 1996.

Marrelli, T.M. *Handbook of Home Health Standards and Documentation Guidelines for Reimbursement,* 2nd ed. St. Louis: Mosby-Year Book, Inc., 1994.

Mastering Documentation. Springhouse, Pa.: Springhouse Corp., 1995.

Milone-Nuzzo, P. "Recognizing and Meeting the Special Needs of Elderly Patients," *Home Health Professional.* Springhouse, Pa.: Springhouse Corp., Winter 1996.

Morgan, K. and McClain, S. *Core Curriculum for Home Health Care Nursing.* Gaithersburg, Md.: Aspen Publishing, 1995.

Nurse's Handbook of Home Infusion Therapy. Springhouse, Pa.: Springhouse Corp., 1997.

Nurse's Legal Handbook, 3rd ed. Springhouse, Pa.: Springhouse Corp., 1996.

Selected references

PharmFacts for Nurses. Springhouse, Pa.: Springhouse Corp., 1996.

Pocket Companion for Home Health Nurses. Springhouse, Pa.: Springhouse Corp., 1997.

Reif, L. and Martin, K. *Nurses and Consumers: Partners in Assuring Quality Care in the Home.* Washington, D.C.: American Nurses Publishing, 1995.

Rice, R. *Home Health Nursing Practice: Concepts and Application,* 2nd ed., St. Louis: Mosby–Year Book, Inc., 1995.

Smith, C.M. and Mauer, F. *Community Health Nursing: Theory and Practice.* Philadelphia: W.B. Saunders Company, 1995.

Teaching Aids for Home Care Nurses. Springhouse, Pa.: Springhouse Corp., 1995.

Index